PU

YOURSELF

FIRST

A busy woman's guide to thriving NOT surviving

Marianne Killick

First printed in 2020 by:
Book Printing UK

ISBN: 978-1-913284-20-6

Printed and bound in Great Britain by:
Book Printing UK Remus House, Coltsfoot Drive,
Woodston,
Peterborough PE2 9BF

ABOUT THE AUTHOR

Marianne Killick (MSc, BA (Hons), PGDipAc, WHC) is a Women's Health Coach and Professional Acupuncturist. Marianne believes that every woman has the right to feel well, to feel empowered in her own body and mind. Marianne's coaching integrates her knowledge of evidence-based medical research on lifestyle medicine, behaviour change and whole-person traditional Chinese Medicine approach to health.

Marianne has spent a decade working with women struggling with issues of hormonal balance, stress, fatigue, fertility issues, PCOS and endometriosis. She has worked with teenagers through to the very elderly and has seen first-hand how the way we live our lives impacts on our hormonal balance and our ability to live well and to thrive. She has helped women to transform their health and their lives to achieve their goals; be that starting a family, living without pain or feeling well enough to take on new professional challenges.

Combined with her own experiences of being a woman trying to balance work and family-life, facing her own health challenges and being part of a women's business community, Marianne has unique insight into not only women's health needs but the struggles they face in daily life when it comes to prioritising their health needs.

After ten years working with victims of torture, Marianne undertook a three year full-time postgraduate level course in acupuncture at the Northern College of Acupuncture in York and is a full member of the British Acupuncture Council.

Marianne is also a graduate of the Integrative Women's Health Institute's Women's Health Coach Certification programme, the only ICHWC internationally approved program for women's health specialists. Marianne is a member of the British Society of Lifestyle Medicine. Marianne is also a speaker and delivers workshops and online courses.

Praise for Put Yourself First

"Put Yourself First is the book that every busy woman needs! While you might have heard that self-care is not selfish, you probably still feel guilty about taking time, energy, or money to take care of yourself. This book is so brilliant because it shows you exactly HOW - with specific ACTION steps - to add self care into your life easily and without guilt. It's easy to say that you need to take better care of yourself, or finally put yourself back on your list, but it can be very hard to put it into practice. This book is the practical guide that you've been looking for. Self-care is not just about manicures and massages, it's a complete lifestyle that's really the secret sauce to productivity. Grab this book, read it this week, and start taking the actions that Marianne maps out... you'll feel better by the end of the week!"
Dr. Jessica Drummond
DCN, CCN, PT, author of Outsmart Endometriosis
Founder and CEO, The Integrative Women's Health Institute

"Put Yourself First is a must read for any women out there with goals and dreams! We all know we are meant to look after ourselves but often the reality of life gets in the way. This book breaks down how to work around that reality of juggling work or running your own business and family life with actually prioritising your own health and well-being so your goals are achievable. There's so much information about how our female bodies work that women just don't know, this book explains to women what's actually happening with their health and hormones in their daily lives so that they can be fully empowered to understand how the choices they make are affecting them. Put Yourself First helps women take their power back. Read it now, take action, so you can go get the life you've always wanted."
Jo Bevilacqua
Founder of The Unique Mumpreneur, multi-award winning entrepreneur and business mentor

For M & A.
May you thrive.

FOREWORD:

Read this book if:

1. You are a woman trying to juggle numerous responsibilities.

2. If you feel tired, stressed, overwhelmed or are just lacking in joy.

3. If you aren't happy with your current state of fitness or health.

4. If you struggle with PMS, hormonal balance, conditions such as PCOS, endometriosis, or want to conceive. Or are heading towards the peri-menopause.

5. If you want to understand how the actions we take on a daily basis directly impact our hormones and what to do about it.

6. If you want help to structure your days more effectively so you have time to do the things YOU want to do.

7. If you need to work on your self-belief and self-worth.

Ask yourself the following questions and take a few minutes to really think about each one:

1. What do I want my health and my life to look like in one, five or ten years time?

2. If I carry on the way i am now, what will my health and life look like in one, five or ten years time?

3. If I make changes that are realistic and totally achievable now, what will my life look like in one, five or ten years time?

Now you are ready to read the book.

TABLE OF CONTENTS

INTRODUCTION:

You First.

Yes, really.

What are your goals? What are your dreams? It doesn't matter. Because, unless you put YOU first, you're unlikely to achieve them.

Think about it:

> The woman with the goal to set up an award winning company...won't get there if she becomes unwell from burnout.
>
> The woman who wants to work part-time and be there equally for her children...won't get there if she hasn't learnt to be fully present instead of stressing about all she has to do and juggle.
>
> The woman who wants to be a stay at home mum and be able to nurture and give all day, every day...won't get there if her own needs aren't met and she's shouty and frazzled.

This isn't about being selfish.

It's about making sure you not only survive, but thrive. But frankly, survival comes into it too. If you don't put you first, look after yourself physically and emotionally, the array of health conditions that await are really rather scary.

It's not about "when the kids have left home I'll look after myself then.." or "once I've got that promotion I'll join the gym", because life has a habit of keeping the obstacles coming.

It's about learning that you are important, that you matter, you matter enough to be prioritised in a world that is ever busier.

And that can be hard to get your head around. As women we are taught that our role is often one of self-sacrifice. That by putting ourselves last, we are benefitting others. I argue that by putting ourselves first we have much more to give others and ourselves. If you are as well rested, well nourished, not stressed out your head, hormonally balanced, think what you could achieve?

So why this book? Why now?

After more or less burning out in my old job, which was high pressured and emotionally demanding, I retrained as an acupuncturist, where for the last decade, I have been seeing men and women, but especially women, doing to themselves what I used to do.

Putting something – *anything*, before self-care.

Then along came the kids and the plan to be a "calm, present, non-shouty nurturing parent" whilst building my acupuncture practice. And being a good loving wife, dutiful daughter, supportive sister, good friend and fit and healthy and zen-like and BANG!

I hit the wall.

So in an effort to create more space to fit it all in I dropped the things that were actually keeping me going; Exercise. Reading for pleasure. Time with friends.

And for a short while it worked, allowed me to catch my breath. But I wasn't fulfilled. Not joyful. Just making space to get by.

And gain 28lbs.

I knew I needed to find more balance, after all, I knew the theory of that, and indeed spend many hours successfully advising people on how to achieve less stress, more balance, lifestyle changes to improve their health.

So why wasn't it working for me? I knew all the information I needed from hours of reading, I was great at motivating others to make changes in their lives, and whilst I was doing great in some aspects of looking after myself, that sense of balance was lacking.

And then whilst training as a women's health coach, it hit me.

All the people coming to see me were being given permission to put themselves first.

To prioritise themselves in a way nobody had encouraged them to do before, rather than treating their own health or emotional needs as an after thought and something to get round to once all the proper jobs are done.

Nobody had given me that permission.

Time to do it for myself. Radical self-care is the name of the game, by which I don't mean spending the whole time being pampered or removing yourself to a remote island. It's taking ourselves back to the basics, backed up by modern research and science.

This book is designed to get you to give yourself that permission to put yourself first. It's designed to give you what you need to know to identify and implement realistic achievable changes specific to you and your life, that won't turn you into an Instagram model but will allow you to achieve a greater sense of calm, more energy and the chance to fulfil your goals.

It won't stop the stuff of life coming at you, but it will help you be better placed to get through it.

I have spent hours reading the latest research on health and well-being. And I have spent years steeped in the ancient Chinese Medicine concept of *Yang Sheng*, or "nurturing life." The ancient Chinese really got the concept of what we today call *Lifestyle Medicine*. The basic idea is that we are born with certain constitutional strengths and weaknesses (our genes) and then it is by how we eat, work or live we either nurture ourselves to live a rich and fulfilling life, or deplete ourselves with stress, poor diet and overwork and fall into illness and trigger disease (epigenetics).

This is not a one-size fits all kind of suggestion list, but a tool to empower you to do what deep down, you probably already know you need to do.

Crucially, this book is also intended to inspire you to know and understand more about how your amazing female body works. If you understand this, you can make better decisions about what's right for *YOU* in your life – not just what you are told is the way to go.

For those inspired to read more or dive deeper into any of the topics raised in this book, there is also a great list of resources to draw from.

When you try to implement the changes you choose after reading this book, it's not necessarily going to fall into place all in one go. You might do really well at getting to bed earlier, but the whole house ends up in chaos. Don't worry. Keep going. The better you get the basics right, good sleep, good nourishment, good movement, over time you'll feel energised enough to work on the rest. When it all falls apart and goes a bit wrong, just re-start, don't waste time on beating yourself up.

You may be already doing some or all of the things suggested in this book, and if so, I salute you. But it never hurts to remind ourselves to stop and take stock of where we are at. Our lives are constantly changing and evolving, and so are our needs and challenges and those of our families, so constant reflection and revision as to what works for you are part of adapting as we grow.

Above all, get excited about the ideas and challenges this book presents to you. As a wise person once said, happiness is not the destination, but the journey. Enjoy opening your mind to the possibility of transformation, enjoying learning more about yourself and trying new ideas. Joy is to be found in the here and now, not at some undefined point in the future.

> *"Beware of destination addiction: The idea that happiness is in the next place, the next job, or even with the next partner. Until you give up the idea that happiness is somewhere else, it will never be where you are."* Robert Holden.

CHAPTER 1: GIVING YOURSELF PERMISSION TO BE A PRIORITY

As women, we are imbibed in a culture of self-sacrifice. I've seen odes to the martyrdom of women praising the woman who sacrifices all in the name of being a "mother". Comments along the lines of "Yes, I'm exhausted, but it's what we do to keep them happy."

I don't think this is entirely healthy. Not on a daily basis.

Of course, in any sort of emergency, we put our children first. But in the course of an average week, most of us are not living in that kind of state of emergency. Historically, it's been incredibly convenient for women to be cast in this role, the role of nurturer, the devoted all-giving super-mum.

Is it our role to keep everyone happy? I believe if we have chosen to have children, it's our role to provide a safe, loving environment that gives our children structure, physical and emotional security, nourishing food and models of positive behaviour. Over time, this equips them with the physical, mental and emotional tools to go out into the world as well-rounded functional adults.

It is not our role to be their maid-servants, to meet their every desire and whim.

I don't believe it's healthy to model always saying yes when you want to say no. Or working yourself to the point of exhaustion. Or break down.

What lessons are we teaching them if they watch us, (and they do watch our every move) become more and more unhealthy, more stressed out and not live a thriving well-balanced life of our own?

If you're reading this and you don't have children, substitute the word *mother* for *wife/partner/daughter*. It all follows the same principle.

Aren't we entitled to live in a way that also meets our own needs? Next time you snap at your kids or partner, or feel frustrated, angry or overwhelmed ask yourself this question: *Which of my needs are not being met?*

Because we all do have needs.

There's plenty of literature out there about the basic needs of a human being. Food, sleep and shelter are the very basics. But to thrive and not just survive, we need community, a sense of connection (sometimes we just need a hug!), a sense of purpose, emotional and spiritual nourishment. *We need physical and mental health to be a priority not an afterthought.*

"You cannot pour from an empty cup."

My argument is this: If we take the time to craft a life for ourselves whereby some re-adjustments of how we structure our day, of how we take on tasks, of how we prioritise our to do lists, so that more of the time most of our needs are being met, will we not be more able to be who we want to be for ourselves and those around us?

If we get the basics of looking after ourselves right, how many of our health issues will we overcome, or prevent happening in the first place? If we get the basics right, how many goals – both personal and professional will we be more likely to meet? How much more likely is it that we will have a happy relaxed home environment?

None of us can prevent tough times coming our way as we go through life, but we can be better placed to handle them. And even with the best plans, there will be events and times where everything gets blown out the water, but having the right mindset and tools to fall back on when you are ready and able to get back on track will be invaluable.

When I see women on my treatment couch who are in pain, in poor health, feeling sad, anxious or at a turning point in their life where they aren't happy, but they don't know how to fix it, I've started asking myself and them, what was their journey to this point? Often there's at least one of the following in the mix:

- Years of caring for another person(s); be that a child, an elderly/sick parent or a spouse
- Lots of stress, either work-place, within their partner relationship or about a child/parent or financial
- Emotional trauma: a bereavement, an abusive parent or partner, pregnancy loss/fertility struggles or other family crisis (addiction/suicide/self-harm)
- Years of not eating food that is doing them any good (the majority of people don't realise what the food industry has done to the nation's health)

9

- A lack of understanding of how their bodies and hormones work (understandable, we aren't actually taught this in school at any point)
- Lack of sleep/lack of *quality* sleep
- Unrelenting exhaustion from dealing with the above
- Years on medication that is doing them more harm than good
- A loss of sense of purpose or direction (particularly for those whose entire identity was as a mother, but the kids have now left home and they aren't yet a grandparent)
- A sense that somehow they are a failure or not good enough for finding life hard, after all, other people have it worse and you just have to get on with it don't you?
- A disconnect between understanding how all of the above impacts on their current physical and emotional health.

In brief, year after year, these women's needs have not been met. If more of us were able to put ourselves first in terms of sleep, nourishing ourselves, understanding our bodies, being aware of our own needs, had better support in place, wouldn't we be more likely to avoid ending up unwell and/or unhappy? If we did even a fraction of what we do for our families for ourselves, we would be more productive, healthier, happier, more at peace. Less overwhelmed.

"Self-care is how you take your power back." (Lalah Delia)

STOP BEING SO HARD ON YOURSELF!

The way most of us talk to ourselves in our heads is not how we would ever talk to someone we cared about or love. We are unrelentingly hard and critical.

> *"Talk to yourself like you would talk to someone you love."* [i] Brene Brown

Too often women have sat in front of me crying with tears of shame and frustration saying "I feel so foolish for not being able to cope with all of this when other people have it *so much worse!*"

Let's take at look at this. Different people are able to cope with different life events and problems in different ways. Why? For a start, we aren't all starting from the same point.

We are all unique. We have different genes, our mother's and grandmother's (yes your grandmother, the egg that made you first came into being when your mother was developing as a baby in her uterus) emotions, life experiences, diet, environment all impact your health and resilience.

Then there was the time, environment and family you were born into. The politics and thinking of the time, your own unique family dynamics, the combination of emotional input from the adults in your life, the comments teachers made to you at school, your friendships, key events in your life, the diet you were fed, the images you saw on television, the good events that happened to you, the bad, whether you were raised to lock feelings away or express them. The medical treatment you received, the kind of birth you had, whether your children slept.

All of these things and many *many* more feed in to make you who you are today. Some of it we've had no say in and no control over whatsoever. Some of it we have. We are constantly evolving works in progress. *We are never finished or complete.*

But crucially all of us are able to do something. Work on our own health and self-development. Our personal growth.

For some, this has to start with recognition that we need to make changes. Others are more ready to leap in with both feet. Wherever you are on that spectrum, that's ok. The fact you are even reading this is a great place to start.

A COFFEE CUP OF SELF-KINDNESS

Imagine you are meeting up with a dear friend you've not seen for a few years. You go for a coffee and you ask them how they are and what's been going on for them since you last saw them. Imagine they tell you all the things that have actually happened in your own life in the last five years.

Now close your eyes and imagine all of that coming out of their mouth. Now ask yourself this, what would you actually say to them in response? Would you be judgemental? Would you be critical? Would you think it was all their own fault?

I'm guessing the answer is no! So please, *don't be so hard on yourself.*

ACTION: make a list of all the things you've found tough, draining or hard in the last five years. Get someone else to read it back to you. Or if you'd prefer, read it out loud to yourself. Now write down all things you would say to someone who told you those things.

Are you crying yet? If you are, it's not surprising. Chances are you've had to deal with a lot the last few years. *You owe yourself a large helping of compassion.*

RECOGNISING THE GREATNESS WITHIN: Celebrating the wonder of you!

Now most of us are appallingly mortified when asked to list our qualities or achievements. It's just not what we do, we might seem big-headed or too proud. We feel self-conscious or foolish. So allow me to help you out! Here are some things you may have achieved in the last few years and here's what they show:

- You may have got a promotion at work: *you worked hard and didn't give up, maybe you pushed yourself out your comfort zone*
- You quit a job you hated: *you showed courage and stood up for yourself*
- You got engaged or married: *you committed to something that meant a lot to you*
- You broke up from someone that wasn't making you happy: *you showed courage to make a leap*
- You quit smoking: *you showed resilience and mental toughness and determination*

- You took up exercise: *you showed determination, openness to challenge, staying power*
- You bought a house: *you showed self-discipline in saving up, organisational skills in getting on top of your finances*
- You got a child to school age: *you've shown love, compassion, tolerance, teaching skills*
- You supported a child through big exams: *you've been solid, an encourager, a cheerleader, a counsellor, a shoulder to cry on.*
- You supported someone through a health crisis: *you've been strong, you've been loving and caring and shown practical and organisational skills*
- You've survived a health crisis: *you've learned when to rest, what your body needs, how to ask for help*

Do you get it? We are all full of greatness when we take a moment to think about it. You deserve to celebrate the great stuff you do and just because some of it is part of daily life as opposed to the stuff of headlines or world records, doesn't make it any less of an achievement.

ACTION: Make your own list of achievements from your life or the last few years and write down the positive things that they say about you. At the bottom of it, write this: I'm AMAZING!

Now, having looked at how far you've come and the things you've already achieved, can you see? You owe it to yourself to put yourself first.

CHAPTER 2: OVERCOMING BARRIERS TO PUTTING YOURSELF FIRST

TIME

Tick tock......

One of the biggest barriers to making healthy changes in life is the belief that there is not enough time. And yes, life does seem to be phenomenally busy these days. It's a class act of juggling work, house and family with *our own needs.*

Was it always this busy? Or is there a culprit?

I think there are several key issues: women are now wanting and trying to do more but their tasks haven't reduced (see the chapter on delegation). Ponder this:

"Even today, around the globe, with so many women in the paid labour force, women still spend at least twice as much time as men doing housework and childcare, sometimes much more. One study of 32 families in Los Angeles found that the uninterrupted leisure time of most mothers lasted, on average, no more than 10 minutes at a stretch. And in mapping the daily lives of academics, the sociologist Joya Misra and her colleagues found that the work days of the female professors were much longer than their male colleagues, once you factored in all their unpaid labour at home. Even so, she found that the men and women she studied spent around the same amount of time at their paid work. But the women's time at work, too, was interrupted and fragmented, chopped up with

more service work, mentoring and teaching. The men spent more of their work days in long stretches of uninterrupted time to think, research, write, create and publish to make their names, and are their careers and get their ideas out into the world." [ii]

We now all spend hours on social media. Have you ever looked at the hours you spend on social media each day? In 2018, the average use was 154 minutes a day! That's crazy! 2 hours and 34 minutes!!! [iii]

But worse than this is our lack of focus. Studies show we look at our screen every twelve minutes [iv]. How can we expect to get anything done? No wonder so many of us now struggle to have a hobby, attend clubs, do exercise, find time to cook healthy meals etc.

Accepting that to keep up with social norms, we are going to be spending some time on social media, let's focus on reducing that time, but also on *working smarter.*

Out of each 24 hour period, 8 of them should be in bed (see chapter on sleep). That leaves 16 hours. Factor in another 8 hours for a job, add on commuting time of roughly an hour each way. That leaves 6 hours in which to do everything else: cook, clean, shower, dress, play with the kids, tend to the kids, shop, laundry etc.

Of course everyone's life and work/life pattern is slightly different. But roughly speaking, could one of those hours could be *just for you?*

The key to fitting everything you want to do in is *planning*. A detailed weekly and daily plan. Most health resolutions or good intentions fail because people don't take the time to sit down, find the time to do the new habit/activity, and don't plan for or anticipate all the things that could derail them.

If you are going to try and fit something new into your life and hope it will become a habit, you need to work out where and how your can do it and have an answer for all the things that will stop you.

ACTION: Turn to the 24 hour planner on page 38. Take a highlighter for sleep, one for hours in work, one for tasks such as cooking etc, one for school run etc. Colour in the 24hour spaces. Now take a different colour and spot the gaps where you could add in exercise or something like reading for pleasure, coffee with a friend.

If, when you do the above task, you are really running out of any space to fit in exercise or relaxation, then please turn to the chapter on delegation and do those exercises.

Remember, if you have a partner, the running of the house and the childcare is *not just your responsibility.*

Think Creatively

It might also be that things can be re-juggled to make space. Are you someone who really wants to fit in a 30min workout in the morning? Can the school lunchboxes be prepared the night before? Can everything be laid out for breakfast in the morning before you sit down for the evening? Could you go to bed 30 minutes earlier and get up 30 minutes earlier?

Start challenging your habits. Just because you've always done something at a certain time of day doesn't mean it can't be shifted. Experiment! What's the worst that could happen?

Can some things be done together? So for example, my favourite way to listen to the health podcasts I want to catch up on are when I'm doing the dishwasher and sorting the kitchen.

Is there more time at weekends to batch cook so you need to spend less time preparing food during the week? Taking two hours to prepare lasagne, shepherd's pie, soup, a curry (all loaded with extra veg!) will pay dividends in the week when you just have to pull portions out the freezer.

Invest in a slow-cooker with a timer. Chuck in the ingredients in the morning and dinner is ready by the time you are home.

Not only is this freeing up time to maybe fit in a work out, planning your business or spending some quality time playing with the kids or supporting homework, it's ensuring you don't resort to processed or junk food.

Can you get your partner to take over some of the duties such as cooking or lunch box prep on some nights? Spread the load. Read the chapter about delegation and planning tasks together! At the risk of repetition; *it's not just your responsibility!*

Schedule Your Day

Are you someone who works from home but the different activities merge and blend together? So in reality there's no clear delineation between anything? You spend the day doing a lot, but feeling like you aren't achieving much?

You would benefit from planning your day, with set times to exercise, do housework, check emails, time to workout, time to shower/dress/makeup. So for example, you might schedule 10am-11am to do housework. Start with the tasks that really need to get done, then move onto the less important ones. Do not check your social media or phone in this time! You'll be amazed at what you can achieve if you don't keep looking at your phone.

At 11am, stop!

This is now your time to do something else you've scheduled that's important. Like respond to emails or focus on your work project. You then get to 12:00 and you may have scheduled 20 minutes to listen to a meditation app, but not all your emails are finished.

Tough, leave them. *There will be time for them later.*

If you don't do the planned meditation, it will be that activity that ends up dropped from the day all together! Treating the scheduled time for your self-care as of equal or greater importance to the other tasks in your day is crucial to *putting yourself first*. It is also helpful to schedule your work-out as your first task, as then it's done.

If it sounds very rigid and rather strict don't be alarmed!

You don't have to plan your whole day this way. Maybe just the time you are at home until you collect the kids from school or until your work shift begins. But if you're feeling pushed for time and overwhelmed at all you have to do - this is an incredibly effective way of getting the most important things done whilst feeling much more in control.

You will need to write a new plan each week or each day, but doing so helps you prioritise around your own daily reality. For example, you may normally work out at 7am every Wednesday, but this week you need to be on the road extra early. Where else can you slot in that work out? If you don't plan when you'll do the activities that benefit your health, *it's fairly guaranteed it just won't happen at all.*

And remember, try doing this exercise with your partner, working out where you can both fit in what you need and want to do.

CHILDCARE:

Another barrier is childcare, especially to exercise.

We hilariously paid for a gym membership and didn't manage to set foot in the gym once. Why? Because one of us has to be in at all times when the kids are home, if the kids aren't home we are working and our working hours don't match up.

By the time we got free time, it was so late in the evening that exercise would have woken us up and frankly, we were too tired.

So the solution has been to look for something we can do without leaving the house.

For us, we have chosen to invest in one piece of equipment: a rowing machine! The monthly payments are cheaper than a gym membership and it's paid off in a year! It's the machine that works the most muscles at once - *working smart is the aim of the game!*

By taking the time to plan our time, and by *adding it at the top of my to do list*, I'm now working out 3-5 times a week. It also doubles as time for headspace.

After a wobbly start, the kids now know that if Mummy is on the rowing machine, they don't interrupt unless someone is hurt or in danger.

They can survive for half-an hour.

This means I get that all important time for thoughts to wander, ideas to form, or just to lose myself thinking about nothing in particular or watching music videos. See the section on setting boundaries to learn more about this.

Or flip it around and use your work-out time to inspire the kids to do the tasks they're not keen on.

One evening, my daughter was protesting the idea of her maths homework, she just wasn't feeling the love! I wasn't feeling like going on the rowing machine. *We made a deal.* If she sat at the table next to the rower and did her homework: I would row. She had to focus to finish her maths before I finished my half-hour row.

We would support each other to get through something we didn't like and we both got our least favourite tasks done and felt good saying "we did it!" The point is this, whether it's a rowing machine or yoga videos, you can find a way around most of the barriers to fitting everything in if you *plan and prioritise activities that put **you** first.* It's the age old adage, *fail to plan: plan to fail.*

And none of this means you can't be spontaneous or just have days where you sack it all off and do nothing. You could limit it to strict scheduling and time slots on just one or two days a week. This is more about giving you a tool to help you see where you can fit in the things that are *important to you without feeling guilty or overwhelmed.* But also to show you that you can be the one in charge of how your time is run, *not the tasks in charge of you.*

Where children can also make it hard to get anything done, like preparing a healthy meal or focusing on a task, is when they are too young for school and their demands are constant and unrelenting.

You've just started preparing food and one of them spills a drink, or needs help on the toilet, or falls over and is crying. By the time you've dealt with everything, the onion you started chopping an hour ago is still in one piece, your mug of coffee is cold and it's almost time to go and collect the older child or get to an appointment.

It's hard, really hard.

But again, *working smart*, especially if you have a partner, is the name of the game.

We have to use the tools we have to help. And yes one of them is the television or iPad. I'm not advocating sticking your child in front of a screen all day, *but use it.* Limit the screen time they get and when they do get it they are more likely to pay attention to it - unlike when it's just constantly on.

Choose a programme they like that is also educational, like Octonauts (anyone else got a child who surprises their nursery teacher with their knowledge of unusual sea-creatures?). In that time, make sure you've planned a task that you can get done, i.e. a quick You-Tube workout, 10 minutes meditation, reading a book you want to read, meal prep, answering your most important work emails etc.

Then when that task is done and the programme is over, spend focussed time *engaged with them* for a bit, talking, interacting. Then maybe do a task whilst they play absorbed alongside you. Or involve them, empty the dishwasher and make a game of them passing you things - it's fun! *They know they have your attention and you are getting a task done.*

Make a game of getting them to help you gather the laundry. Yes, it's a bit slow, but your child feels valued and useful. *They are learning a useful skill: you are giving them attention and achieving a task.*

And importantly, accept the imperfection of life at this time. It won't always be this chaotic and crazy. *Nobody ever died because household tasks weren't done to perfection.*

Divide and conquer with your partner or another family member or friend! Can they be on child duty whilst you spend an hour really focussed on your exercise or meditation? Or the other way around? It's teamwork.

It's more valuable to the child to have your totally undivided attention for a short while than have half your attention whilst you half-ignore them all day. You'll both end up frustrated and grumpy! *You and your partner are likely to get along better if you've both had that downtime to yourself.*

Making life more efficient means there will be more space in that 24 hour period in which to take that time to dedicate to your own health, your own needs. And when you do that, you'll be so much more ready to connect with your child and partner and engage with them in a way that makes *you and them happy.*

THE MENTAL LOAD:

Another aspect of not enough time is just how full our brains are. Studies show that despite an improvement in the sharing of domestic tasks since women went out to work more, the mental load is still carried by the woman.[v]

Women are not only working, and parenting, but also being an *overall general and domestic manager.* How many of us are the ones who as well as running our own job/business, keep on top of who is growing out of what, needs new shoes, reply to party invites, make sure presents and cards are bought, plan birthday parties, organise Christmas, stay on top of everyone's dental/optician appointments, school trips, keeping in touch with other relatives, pet care, paying bills, booking the holiday?.....I could go on.

Sometimes, it's also about more than just having physical time to do stuff. Many of us are mentally exhausted and the idea then of trying to change eating habits or implement a new exercise plan is frankly just one more thing too far.

Again, apart from learning to delegate and making a point of asking our partners to take charge of certain things like buying presents for their own family members, taking the time to write a list of everything that needs to happen can be incredibly cathartic.

You may need more than one list! A list of things to happen for your child's party, for Christmas present buying, food ordering, holiday prep, work to do lists. Work project to do lists. Making lists keeps things ordered and in control and is *a relief for your brain to dump it all onto paper*. And then *delegate as much of it as you can.*

But more important still, is the importance of *prioritising doing nothing.*

Schedule it if you have to: 20 mins coffee break. But make sure you use it for sitting with your coffee relaxing, staring into space or if you can't sit still doing nothing, doing something you want to do: read a book, knit, crotchet, paint, meditate. Something where you can lose yourself into thought that wanders.

Not only is this decompression for the mental pressures we feel, but it actually helps us problem solve. How often have you come up with your best ideas when standing under the shower with your mind wandering? Taking time to just be is incredibly important for creative thinking, and is something that the likes of Einstein and Darwin did as a matter of routine, spending time lost in thought.[vi]

It's ok to do nothing. I'll repeat that again. It's ok, in fact, essential to your well-being to *spend time doing nothing*. Forget this culture of being busy that we seem to be glamourising. Be a rebel and turn up somewhere and instead of saying "Oh my gosh I've got so much on!" Say, "Hey, yes I've got lots to do when it's scheduled to be done, *but right now I'm doing nothing!*"

The ancient Chinese had a similar but slightly different slant on doing nothing. Something called the art of *Wu Wei*, or "non-action". Broadly speaking, this doesn't mean sitting around doing nothing at all, but more *doing things in-line with the natural flow of life.*

Not fighting against what we feel we ought to be doing. Doing things in a way that we are in harmony and in a flow state *where things happen and get done without strain or struggle.*

I translate this into two different things. Being in flow state is where you are totally immersed in what you are doing in the moment, and what you need to do just comes naturally and instinctively. And listening to your body and mind.

An example of flow state is when I'm fully present and immersed with my patients in my acupuncture clinic. It's not an effort or hard for me to know what to do. My knowledge, my learning and instinct come together and allow me to treat the patient.

For an artist, they don't need to think how to paint the curve of a flower-petal, they are "in the zone" and it comes naturally. When you knit, you don't need to think what to do next, your fingers just move instinctively to twist and loop the wool.

When we achieve this flow state, we don't feel frazzled and frantic - but calm and not depleted. We can try and create this flow state in our work by having clear systems and procedures in place, in our home by having structure and routine. And when we are relaxing, by losing ourselves in something pleasurable, whatever that may be for you.

The second aspect is not fighting the natural flow of life. So, on days when we really just don't have the energy or are too mentally exhausted, permitting ourselves to not fight it and to take the time to rest.

As women, where we have a cycle that ebbs and flows with different energies and feelings. It's particularly important that we don't try too hard to fight against what our body is telling us. This is something that will be covered in more detail in the chapter about your hormones and body.

If nothing else, let's ensure we let our children have time to just be.

Sometimes, we need to say no to the crazy number of activities they can be involved in and give them time just to be. Playing at home in their rooms or the garden with nothing but free time to let them drift and wander into fantasy land. It's important for their mental health, their creativity and their brain-connections.

Again, this is where if you're still wondering how you can justify this time out to yourself, *you can use this to model balance to your children.*

> *"No is a necessary magic. No draws a circle around you with chalk and says "I have given enough."* (McKayla Robbin)

YOU as a barrier:

One of the biggest barriers to making changes in our lives is *ourselves.*

We tell ourselves so many stories that simply aren't true but we never dare think to question them! How often do we say things like "Well I just can't fit any more in?" Or "I'm just not someone who can ever be slim!" Or, "I'm no good at cooking/sport/hairstyling…", "All the women in my family are overweight, it's just how we are!" We talk ourselves out of change before we even try!

We also assume that unless we can do things perfectly then we may as well not bother. How about a new mantra in life: *"Not perfect, but done."*

- A 30 min jog where we walked for half of it as we're still building up fitness is way better for us than not going at all because we know we can't run the full half-hour.
- Ten minutes trying to meditate but achieving peace for only 2 mins is much better than nothing at all.
- A meal with extra veggies and a defrosted "here's one I made earlier" is better than ordering a take-away.
- Losing 5lbs but still having 30 to go is better than not losing any.

Again, *stop being so hard on yourself* - trying and *getting it half-done is better than not trying at all*. Each small effort you make is helping you towards better health and well-being.

We also assume people are judging us or will judge us if we do things differently. And you know what, they might! Some will be full of admiration for any positive changes you make. Some will criticise you and knock you down as you changing holds a mirror up to their own lives and their lack of change. It's much easier to tear someone else down than look at yourself!

You might get told you're being too strict, you're stressing yourself out, or in tones that denote anything but approval, "you've CHANGED!" Heavens forbid!

Once you set upon a course of action, *it's so important to surround yourself with people who have your back.* Occasionally, you laying down some boundaries and becoming focused is just too much for some people. But those who get that you're trying to look after yourself so you can be the best version of you will be your champions.

> *"A shark in a fish tank will grow 8 inches, but in the ocean it will grow to 8 feet or more. The shark will never outgrow its own environment and the same is true about you. Many times we're around small thinking people so we don't grow. Change your environment and watch your growth."* (Bob Harrison)

Those who are part of a community striving towards the same thing are more likely to succeed in their goals. That community can be an organised group, or just you and your bestie striving to make similar changes.[vii]

THE THOUGHTS IN OUR HEADS

> *"What you think, you become. What you feel, you attract. What you imagine, you create."* Buddha

It's important to understand that what we spend our times telling ourselves is what becomes our reality.

So if we spend our time telling ourselves we're fat, we're just someone who isn't sporty, or we have hormonal issues that can't be changed, then it will be so.

Here's a few examples of common limiting beliefs:

> I'm not smart enough
> I can't start, I'm not ready

I'm a mess, it's hopeless
I don't have enough time
I'm so unhealthy there's too much work to do
Change is too hard
I just have bad luck
I'm not self-disciplined
I don't have as much money as X who got healthy

Our brains are fundamentally lazy, and choose the easiest thought path. The easiest thought paths are the ones that have been most trodden. *So if we want to change we have to tread a new path so eventually it becomes our brain's quickest route.*

This is where when people talk about "manifesting" or "*mental rehearsal*", the idea of visualising the reality we want for ourselves comes in. Our brains aren't able to distinguish our imagined future from our current reality. Athletes use this in their training, visualising their win.[viii]

Visualise yourself coming last and guess what will happen? The power of our mind is in fact so great that we can actually change biological markers by thought alone[ix]. So if we want to create a new reality for ourselves then we need to be clear what that is and spend time each day visualising ourselves as that person.

This may sound like hocus pocus, but the neuroscientist Dr Joe Dispenza spends his time studying and training people in exactly this. It's not something that will take effect in just one go, but day after day of practise and it will filter through into your behaviour. Meditation works along the same principles and has been shown to change brains within relatively short periods of time.

ACTION: Pick an aspect of your health that you want to improve. For example, having a healthy waist measurement. Close your eyes and picture yourself looking like you will once you've met your goal. Visualise how you feel, how your body feels when you move, how clothes feel on your body. What is your mood like in this vision? Imagine yourself walking down the street and meeting people you know, how does it feel? Visualise yourself doing activities like dancing or hiking with this new healthy body. How are you feeling? Do this every night for a week and notice how it gradually impacts your daily choices.

Repeating affirmations is another popular way of getting us to follow through on our deepest desires. It's not so much a question of "fake it 'til you make it" but "repeat it 'til you live it." Again, it's training your brain to have new thought pathways. *Drumming in a positive message.*

After all, the negative thoughts we have had instilled in us and the limiting beliefs are something we've had drummed into us by (sometimes well-meaning) adults who raised us, the society we are in and by ourselves. Look how effective they've been at holding us back and keeping us stuck! If we think how powerful these have been for negative outcomes think what turning them on their head could do! *If your thoughts are limiting, so will your behaviour be.*

ACTION: Pick a limiting belief, maybe something like "I'm rubbish at doing exercise, i get it all wrong and just give up,

I'm useless." Now try flipping it around: "I am great at moving my body for my health, I feel fantastic when I do it! I'm winning at getting fitter! " Or how about swapping "it's more important to look after the needs of the family than my own" with "when I care for myself first, my family does even better!" Write them out on a piece of paper. Stick them where you will see them every morning, repeat them every morning. You'll feel fake and a right idiot the first few times you do this but persevere. Repeat it when sat at traffic lights. Notice how energised you feel when you focus on this positive affirmation. Amazing right?

Having the belief that you as you are today are *not the finished product*, and that you are capable of growth, development and *change is crucial* to your success at reaching whatever goals you have in life.

Working on your mindset is crucially important and I can't recommend Dr Carol Dweck's work on this highly enough[x]. She gives example after example how those who can twist any setback into a learning experience to grow from, those who believe they can always improve, those who spend time working on themselves not in competition with others, those who don't just blame circumstance or others for their failures, are the ones to transform their lives and not only be successful, but feel *successful and accomplished.*

This is true as much in our *personal lives* as in our *professional lives*, and is crucial to understand in terms of giving our children a growth mindset for life.

As you start to truly believe you can be the *best version of yourself* that you can be, it will become easier to change some of our less healthy habits and to prioritise your own self-care.

> *"Even with the knowledge and tools to become healthier, happier individuals, it is often our mindset and daily practices that will be the strongest guiding force to carry us through our health journey."* Dr Mark Hyman

Belief that you can be the person you want to be and that you are *worthy of prioritising this is paramount* to helping you stick with it when the going gets tough. But first you may need to identify not only the vision of the life you want, or the health you want, but your reason behind it!

If you don't know your goals, and the reasons behind them, your chances of sticking to new routines or picking yourself up when you face obstacles are severely reduced.

KNOWING OUR "WHY?"

> *"When you have nothing to aim at, you have no reason to organise and master yourself. No goals, no growth. No clarity, no change. Let ambition swell in your heart once more. Set your own course."* Brendon Burchard

One of the best ways to ensure we follow health-giving behaviours and to prioritise them is to do it for a reason that has a greater purpose than merely being healthy. Research shows that people who have meaning and purpose are more effective at what they are doing when that purpose is for something outside of themselves.[xi]

In fact Esfahani-Smith describes that meaning in life is comprised of four pillars: belonging, purpose, story-telling and transcendence[xii]. To summarise, if you have a sense of being part of community, be that your family, a friendship group, social community or your work community, your meaning comes from the contribution you feel you are making to the lives of those amongst whom you belong.

Your purpose comes from contributing to the greater good of the world in which you live, be that through doing the dishes to help your home life run smoothly or finding a cure for a major disease. If you have a sense that what you're doing is for the benefit of others or the greater good your life will be more satisfying. *The more likely you'll put more effort into what you do.*

If the narrative you tell yourself about your life is one that looks for the meaning and strengths and passions to come out of past sufferings you will have a greater sense of meaning. If you realise you are just one tiny part of something way bigger and more precious than ourselves you will be driven to work for something bigger than yourself.

At first sight, this all sits at odds with the title of this book, *Put Yourself First*. But as per my introduction, it's not intended to be about me me me. It's all about allowing us to be in the best place possible to fulfil our sense of purpose and contribute to those around us and so that we are as well and as healthy as possible so as to be able to exercise the right to choose how we spend our time and our days, not have it decided for us by the state of our health. *It's so you are healthy and well enough to live the life of meaning that you wish to live.*

For each of us, that purpose and meaning will be different. My meaning comes from being part of my family, wanting to live a life that sets a good example to my children to give them the foundation to live their dreams, whatever they may be.

I want to work on my health and fitness so I can be the Mummy I aspire to be and so I can share new experiences with my children as they get older. I don't want to succumb to diabetes as my grandmother did, because she was from a time where women came last and medical care wasn't where it is now.

I want to feel energetic and healthy so I can achieve my ambitions to empower as many women as possible in their self-care. I feel strongly that my journey through my own struggles and then the experiences in my clinic give me knowledge I want to share for the benefit of other women out there who just aren't being taught what they need to know to thrive.

ACTION: Take the time to reflect on what has brought you to where you are now and how it's taught you important lessons, skills and strengths or given you a mission. Think about who your actions impact and how you feel you contribute to the lives of those around you, not necessarily in big dramatic ways, but even in smaller more subtle ways. What would you like to achieve in this life? What message have you got to share? What difference do you want to have make? Think about what makes you want to

get up each day and how being healthy and well-rested and nourished will help you achieve your dreams, whatever they are.

There are no dreams or purposes that are better than others. It's all so personal and your dreams and goals might be totally different to those of your friend or your sister. But the one thing they all have in common is their chances of becoming reality if you put your self-care first.

CONCLUSION: You can work all you want on time management and delegation, but if the voice in your head tells you it's not going to happen, or you're not worth it, you are going to struggle. Working on yourself your mindset, your self-belief, your self-awareness and understanding of what makes you tick is fundamental to being courageous enough to put yourself first.

24 HOUR PLANNER

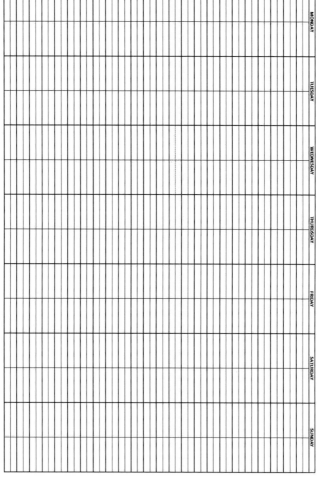

	MONDAY	TUESDAY	WEDNESDAY	THURSDAY	FRIDAY	SATURDAY	SUNDAY
00:00							
01:00							
02:00							
03:00							
04:00							
05:00							
06:00							
07:00							
08:00							
09:00							
10:00							
11:00							
12:00							
13:00							
14:00							
15:00							
16:00							
17:00							
18:00							
19:00							
20:00							
21:00							
22:00							
23:00							

KEY: Colour 1: My Workout/My Meditation/My Do Nothing Time
Colour 3: Work
Colour 5: Sleep

Colour 2: Domestic Tasks (cooking/Cleaning Laundry)/Childcare Tasks (Clubs/Feeding/Changing)
Colour 4: Quality Time with Partner/Kids

Marianne Killick COACHING

38

CHAPTER 3: THE IMPORTANCE OF UNDERSTANDING YOUR HABITS AND ENVIRONMENT

BEING A CREATURE OF HABIT:

Not only do you need to sort your beliefs, sort your vision for what you want and your why, but reflecting on the daily habits that hold us back is crucial.

We are all creatures of habit more than we can ever realise.

Each time we repeat an activity we are creating a feedback loop in our brain until certain things become automatic and are done without thinking. Like raising a cup to our mouth or the actions we take when driving our car. When we look in detail at our lives our days are made up of hundreds, if not thousands of habitual processes.

In fact, *almost half our daily actions are automatic habits.*[xiii] This includes automatically eating left-over food from our children's plate, reaching for a biscuit every evening, pouring that extra glass of wine, or flopping onto the sofa instead of going out for the run you know you meant to do!

In the book *The Power of Habit*, the author explains *The Golden Rule of Habit Change*. Everything we do is broken down into three stages: the cue, the routine, the reward.[xiv]

So the cue might be the time of day, or sitting in a team meeting. The routine might be reaching for cake, the reward is the sugar hit and what you feel when you eat the cake. The craving for the cake is actually your brain jumping ahead and anticipating and wanting the reward as soon as it sees the cue. Once that craving kicks in, it's pretty hard to say no. And it's how marketing works, with smells, or even just the symbol of our favourite fast-food chain making our brain jump ahead and anticipate the reward.

The trick, Duhigg says, is to change the routine. *Replace it with something different.* Such as making and stirring a mug of coffee instead of reaching for the cake. But more than that, you need to understand why you are reaching for the donut in that meeting.

So you need to understand your cue. Is it really that you are hungry? Is it that you are actually nervous, and having something to do with your hands, gives you a sense of purpose and masks your nerves in front of others? Is it that everyone else is doing it and you want to fit in?

And finally, you need to understand the reward you are actually getting: Is it the sugar? Or is it the sense of being part of the team, or is it the safety of your fears being hidden?

Once you start breaking down each of the habits you want to change like this, it becomes so much easier to figure out an *effective replacement* to the routine you no longer wish to do.

ACTION: Pick one habit that you want to change. Break it down into three sections: Cue, Routine, Reward. Now take the time to think about the cue, what's actually going on for you? You might need to spend several days making notes about your particular habit to spot what the issue

actually is. The reward: What is it you are really getting out of it? The routine, what can you swap it for? If you're struggling with this let me share how I approached this with one of my habits:

As far as eating my children's left-overs, no way would I pick at someone else's half-eaten fish finger! But somehow, when it's at home on my children's plate, without thinking, that half-fishfinger finds its way to my mouth. So why can't I stop doing this at home? Let's break it down:

Cue: Seeing left over food on the plate: Am I actually hungry at this point? Sometimes, yes I am. I've prepared the children's food and am planning to have dinner a bit later with my husband. I notice I don't pick so much when I'm also having dinner at the same time as the kids. Also, I struggle to leave an empty plate, I was raised in the era of "clear your plate." So this is triggering my "we mustn't waste food" button and I'm actually feeling a bit annoyed at the thought of throwing food away.

Routine: Eating the left-overs. How can I change this? And what to?

Reward: Tasty food. Is my reward the food? The satiation of hunger? Partly, especially if I'm actually hungry. Or is the reward the satisfaction of nothing going to waste?

So here's my new routine!

Once the kids have their plates of food I start to prepare a small snack, maybe some carrot sticks, a piece of fruit, a few raisins. When the kids have finished their meal **(the cue)**, I start munching my snack **(routine)** then myself or preferably the kids take their plates over to the bin and scrape the leftovers into the composter, and place any scraps of meat or fish into the dog bowl **(routine)**. **The reward** is: I'm satisfied with my snack, there's not much waste going on. And I'm no longer eating so many unnecessary calories.

This is a really good exercise to do, especially around evening snacking or drinking. Really, what is the reward we are seeking? What is the unmet need we are seeking to fulfill? Is it lack of joy, is it not being recognised for our hard work all day, is it boredom or loneliness from lack of deep communication?

It will be different for everyone. Once we start breaking down our habits like this, we get a deeper understanding of what's actually happening for us, and this gives us huge power over what we then do with these unwanted behaviours.

This is one of the areas where working with a health coach can support you in identifying what's actually going on for you. Often we are so lost in our daily habits and routines, it can be hard to isolate patterns and unpick what's behind them.

The *Golden Rule of Habit Change* also works the same when we actually want to start doing something, such as *working out*. We need to *create* a **cue**, such as seeing our trainers by the door, seeing it written on our schedule. The **routine** is the workout. The **reward** is the feel-good at the end, the knowing we are a step closer to our vision, the satisfaction of having done something you find hard and the buzz of feeling energised.

If we train our brain to focus on the **reward** as soon as we see the **cue**, (creating the craving) we will want to do that work out. The hardest part is repeating this new routine often enough to create the craving of the reward as soon as we see the cue.

And this is where supporting our will-power comes in.

Willpower, it has been discovered, is something that if you exert in one area of your life, will automatically filter into other areas. So as you become more disciplined in ensuring you fit that work out in, you are more likely to resist purchasing things you don't need or taking the second cookie.[xv]

It's like a positive cascade effect and it's why some people seem to undergo incredible transformations, like losing 80lbs and also then getting out of debt and studying for the degree they always wanted. They become skilled in exerting their willpower. That combined with their *greater belief in themselves* and their "*why*" is like a *tidal wave of positive change.*

One of the major things you can do to support your willpower is making a *plan*. Studies show that those who write down their goals are much more likely to succeed.[xvi] And it's not simply a question of writing "lose 10lbs," it's *detailing each action* you need to take and what will you do at "pain points" or things you know you are going to struggle with. It comes back to breaking things down and *planning*, planning how you will do something, when and how you will do it and what you will do when you meet obstacles.

Another thing again, is community. A buddy system that makes it more fun to do or at the very least, guilts you into not letting the others down!

UNDERSTANDING YOUR ENVIRONMENT:

> *"When a flower doesn't bloom, you fix the environment in which it grows, not the flower."* (Alexander Den Heijer)

Our self-control, or *willpower*, and ability to override unhealthy choices or create new habits is also directly affected by the situations in which we find ourselves.[xvii]

Studies show that those who make the best choices are not solely relying on conscious decisions and strength of will power, but favourable situations.[xviii] In other words, creating a situation or environment that makes healthy behaviour your default option without having to actually try.

Because knowing what we should be doing is not enough to make us do it. If it were we'd all be Size 8, toned and ace at relaxing and having fun on demand! In other words, if the environment around you supports healthy behaviours your actions will be healthier.

Whole towns can have their health changed by having their environments changed! The National Geographic explorer Dan Buettner believes longevity ensues from the right environment. In his own words *"healthy choice being the only choice is the secret"*

Check out the following statistics[xix]:

- If you live in an area with 6 fast food restaurants within half a kilometre of your house, you are 40% more likely to be obese than if there are fewer than 3.
- If you live in a neighbourhood that has billboards advertising junk food you are 10% more likely to be obese than if there are no billboards.
- If you live in a neighbourhood with bike lanes, pavements and clean parks, you will have physical activity levels 20-30% higher than if you don't.

This is crazy, but it highlights that over and above any kind of active conscious decision-making, the environment around us impacts our health. It's all about what is laid out as an easy option right in front of you!

Big companies create environments that favour you buying their products *without thinking too much about it*. How? They make your life super easy, they make it easy so there are few barriers to buying their products. They create the *cue, routine, reward* behaviours and then take away all your barriers to carrying out the habit.[xx]

Notice how you have to queue for your coffee right in front of the cake counter for several minutes. Then the barista asks you if you want a cake with your coffee. If the cake hadn't been there right in front of you the previous few minutes, your chances of saying no would be higher.

They make your behaviour *"frictionless"*[xxi]: If we do this in our home environment and in our daily workplace, it will be so much easier to make *good healthy choices.* Notice above with the fish-finger example, part of the *new routine* was actually changing my environment; it is no longer me being faced with the fish-finger on the plate as the children are scraping their own plate. It's instantly easier for me not to eat it if it's not in front of me.

In all the Blue Zones, or areas where people live long and healthy that Buettner describes, their surroundings favour healthy behaviours as the *automatic response.*[xxii] From the Chinese Medicine perspective, the whole purpose of living in balance and of *Yang Sheng* or, nurturing life, is to avoid getting sick in the first place! It's far easier to maintain health than to come back from a place of ill-health.

So here's the question, how can you make *your immediate environment favourable* to your desire to put yourself first and make *healthy choices*? Creating routines, expectations and structure as described in the chapters on *barriers to change* and *delegation* is part of it. But so is what you stock in your cupboards, the people you mix with, what you watch, the places you go and so on.

Start asking, if I want to make exercise part of my daily life, as well as creating a new habit as described above, how can I make this *super easy and the only choice?* How can I build activity into my life so it becomes automatic?

If I want to eat more vegetables through the working week, how can I make this *super easy and my default response?* Again your answers need to reflect your reality, your work pattern, and importantly, they need to *come from you* or you are less likely to actually try it out! The following chapters are designed to help you find *your own answers* to these questions.

"Get into the habit of asking yourself, 'Does this support the life I am trying to create?'" wildwomanbusinesshood.com

CHAPTER 4 YOU CAN'T DO IT ALL BY YOURSELF!

The art of delegation.

They say it takes a village to raise a child. I say it takes a village to run your own business or achieve your dreams. And if you want to do both, raise a child and achieve your professional dreams, you need not just a village, but a *well-organised and structured team around you*.

One of the most transformative experiences of recent times for me has been getting involved in the community of *The Unique Mumpreneur*, a supportive group of women all trying to juggle family life with running their own business and reaching their dreams. It's run by the inspirational *Jo Bevilacqua*. One of the first mantras I heard repeated there was – *delegate*. Delegate everything you can!

Get someone else to do what *you don't like or aren't good at*. That way you have more time to dedicate to the things that actually get you closer to your goals and give you more time to spend with those you love. For those of us who struggle to *relinquish control* of aspects of our business or even to admit we can't do it all, this can be a *big leap*.

The other has been the *health coaching* I've undergone as part of my training to become a *women's health coach*. This has taught me to look at what support I have around me, where the gaps are, and to evaluate where I can ask for help and restructure how I live.

And the final big lesson, has been from my acupuncture patients, where I have learnt what happens long-term if you keep trying to pour from an empty cup. I've seen too many women on the treatment couch who have utterly exhausted themselves over decades of trying to be *all things to all people.*

In fact, if I hadn't learnt the art of delegation from all these things there is no way this book would have come into fruition.

ACTION: Here's an exercise I undertook with Jo Bevilacqua on one of her weekend goal setting retreats and if you've ever had any doubts about needing to delegate, i really suggest you do this:

- Grab a big A3 sheet of paper, or a bunch of A4 pages if you don't have one.
- Grab a bunch of coloured pens.
- Allocate a colour to each aspect of your life, your partner, your home, your kids, your job or your business, other family members such as parents etc.
- Write their name in colour in different areas of the sheet. *Don't forget to add yourself.*
- Now brainstorm every single thing you can think of that you need to do daily, weekly, monthly or yearly for each of these things and write them all down around the relevant name.
- Include obligations you already have, dreams you'd like to achieve, goals you'd like to set.

It might take you a little while.

And then when you feel slightly airless and overwhelmed at the sprawling mass of writing you've just created and the sheer scale of what's there in front of you, of all the things you need to do and want to achieve, *BREATHE.*

You've got this.

And this is why you are going to start delegating. *And learning to say no.*

When I did this exercise on the goal-setting retreat, I actually felt I might have a panic attack when I looked at it all. And then *I felt proud at the amount I had achieved already.* You see, most of us are actually *Superwoman already!*

But the mental load of it all can be crippling. And I knew to achieve my goals of being a present mummy, my own health goals and my professional dreams. I had to get over myself as being the only heroine on the page and *enlist some help.*

So start with the things that stress you out the most: for me, it wasn't actually my professional goals, but the state of the house. I was actually embarrassed by the state it was getting in each week as myself and my husband tried to juggle his full-time work, my long days in clinic, obligations to other family members and pets and give quality time to the kids.

In fact, this fell into the category of "what can you delegate that will free you up to do what you love and are good at" because frankly I hate housework! I'm rubbish at it! And it was getting in the way of *quality time with my son*, when I wasn't at work, or getting on with the business of working on my business.

Weekend time was being dominated by trying to get through it all rather than doing fun-stuff. Or spending *quality time together*.

So I followed Jo's advice and got a cleaner.

Instead of getting up on a Friday morning and not only being tired from intense clinic days, but then facing a house in a state, and guilt at the "quality time" I wanted to give to my son being diluted with "in a minute when I've finished cleaning we will do something" was replaced with "yes let's go to the park, visit the farm" and now he's in school, is my time for further study, writing, working on my business, or some days, *just do nothing*.

It's saved my sanity when some days I'm tired, but walk in to an oasis of calm and my bed is beautifully made as if I was in a hotel. *The effect is instant calm*. My fear was affording it. As Jo said, *you can't afford not to*.

Attending *The Unique Mumpreneur* events also opened up a world to me of services and support I never knew existed. I'd heard of a virtual assistant, but never really thought it was something that applied to me. How wrong was I!

I'm awful at anything IT or tech related, slow at creating documents, and a procrastinator for all the stuff I find boring, like doing my spreadsheets. I assumed I had to battle on and slog through it myself, as I was too small to employ someone. No! There exists services like that for people like me! The biggest challenge was trusting someone to not mess it up. But that's also about good communication and really working with the person who is supporting you. I tried a few tasks out with a Virtual Assistant, and found it went well, so gradually added more.

I now have more time to spend researching my patient's medical issues, getting on top of the latest health research, in other words, *doing the stuff I love* that actually makes me good at what I do.

The same principles apply to many jobs, *not just the self-employed*. Are you taking on too many tasks that could be delegated to those around you? Do you have an issue letting go of stuff that's actually weighing you down? Have you asked for more support from your boss? Is there a case for explaining to your boss that the salary you are being paid is better spent on you doing the stuff that is more productive for the company when someone else could be doing tasks better done by an assistant instead?

ACTION: Look at the mind dump you've just done on the previous exercise, now make a list of any of the tasks on there that stress you out the most or that you least enjoy. These are the ones to work on delegating first. Set yourself a date by which you will have enquired and engaged help.

The art of the TO DO List:

It's kind of like a "write down your worries and symbolically burn them" exercise to have a good to do list!

Personally, if I've got it all written down I feel more in control. I always have one in my work bag, and spend time writing a fresh one each week. It also helps me work out each day and each week which tasks I need to delegate and which tasks I'm going to need help from someone else.

But here's an interesting question:

- Where on your daily to-do list is the stuff that relates to your own *well-being?*
- Your physical or mental health?
- Did "exercise" or a "mindfulness app" even make it on there?
- Did read a chapter of the new novel by your favourite author get on there?
- Or book an acupuncture treatment for yourself?
- Or 15 mins *doing nothing?*

It sounds simple, but the act of not only including such things on your to do list, but putting them right at the top is highly significant both in terms of demonstrating repeated commitment to the fact that you deserve to *PUT YOURSELF FIRST,* but also to increase the likelihood of actually doing it.

Since I started doing this, I've actually done more work-outs than I've done in the entirety of my life thus far! It's created a *positive spiral,* I'm more energised because I've worked out, which means I feel more focussed and am more efficient, and because I don't want to lose that feeling and motivation I keep prioritising my self-care. Try it. *PUT YOURSELF FIRST.*

" We need to do a better job of putting ourselves higher on our own 'to do' list." Michelle Obama

Delegating and daily chores at home:

The fact that women are working outside of the home and yet still shouldering the major burden of all household tasks is frankly depressing. In this modern age, there's no excuse for a household not to be a *team effort.* And yet even with the most supportive, enlightened and willing to do their share partners, a lot can *still fall on women*.

It was during a *health coaching* call with my master coach where I was bemoaning how tired I was that we worked on unravelling why I was getting to bed so late. She asked me, "How old is your daughter? Can she not do some of her bag preparation for the next day?" It dawned on me how habits had just formed in our daily lives that *weren't enriching any of us.*

I strongly believe that as a parent, our role is to help raise independent young people to go into the world filled with resourcefulness to tackle whatever challenges and opportunities come their way. The behaviour we model to them as parents will directly shape the expectations of how their own family life should run.

Do we want for our daughters to feel as frazzled as many of us can feel? Do we want our sons to be the kind of husbands or fathers who don't play their part? There's some great studies out there that show how children who take part in the household chores do better at school, are better team players, and have a more resourceful and positive outlook on life[xxiii]. Why? Because they are being *empowered to feel in charge of their own life*, they are getting the buzz of team work and the reward of family time when tasks are done, they are being taught problem-solving and resourcefulness and resilience. Here is a handy chart of age appropriate tasks kids can do:

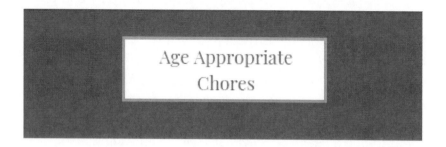

Age Appropriate Chores

AGED 3 AND UNDER	AGED 4 - 6	AGED 7 - 9
Tidy away toys	Set the table	Put away clean clothes
Make bed	Feed pets	Hover / sweep floors
Fold up pyjamas and	Dress themselves	Help prepare food
place on bed	Clear the table	Clean kitchen counters
	Water plants	Empty / fill dishwasher
	Help pair socks	Help put away food
	Make their bed	shopping

AGED 10 -12	AGED 13 +
Empty the bin	Help with siblings
Change their bed	Clean car
Wash-up	Mop floors
Fold washing	Clean bathroom
Walk the dog	Babysit
Help with cooking	Prepare a basic meal

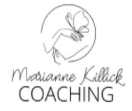

Marianne Killick
COACHING

ACTION: identify what household tasks you alone normally do can sometimes or all the time be done by others in your house.

Maybe you are doing some of these things already, we were. But we hadn't taken the time to re-evaluate every so often as the kids grow, or the weekly structure of school etc changes. Kids understand more than you think.

Explaining that you really want to spend time on the sofa with them watching Harry Potter, but won't be able to if you have to do all the tasks by yourself as you won't get time to sit down can be useful. That you want to take them to all their activities but won't have time to also bake with them this weekend if nobody helps gather the laundry.

It makes them realise helping out is in their own interest. Are they always happy little helpers? Of course not. But having a basic set of expectations and tasks for each child sets a baseline. Having a daily routine of things they have to do. *They get used to it*.

They want you to purchase that extra app for them? Did they do all their basic tasks? No? No app! And when they do what's been asked of them or they surprise you by doing something extra helpful, what a pleasure to do something extra fun with them or surprise them back with an unexpected treat! And how lovely for the *whole house* that no *one person is totally exhausted and snappy*.

And here's one of the key things. *ASKING FOR HELP*.

We all get into our own heads and sometimes our partners can't read our minds. A regular conversation with your partner along the lines of, "so this week I'm working late two nights, you're working late on another, what's our plan this week for getting meals cooked, and getting the laundry ready?" can go a long way.

Going through a *weekly* and *monthly calendar* and planning out together who is going to do what, so it all gets done means *everyone is clear on what needs to happen* and no one person is left shouldering the burden. Sometimes it's essential to spell it out and say: "We can't get where we want to as a family unless we both have some structure and planning as to what needs to get done around the house and for the kids, *it's not working for me how it is right now*." Yes, some weeks it will all fall apart, the house will look like a disaster zone and instead of a healthy home cooked meal you dial a take away. *That's all ok too.*

ACTION: Make a list of tasks that need to happen this next week, sit down with your partner and talk about how as a couple you can get through them all.

If you receive hostility when you do this, then there may be some deeper work to be done on this as a couple. *There's no scope in this book for that kind of couple counselling*. But as a starting point, there are some names of organisations in the Further Help and Resources section.

Learning to say NO and creating healthy boundaries:

> "*Love yourself enough to create boundaries. Your time and energy are precious. You get to choose how you use it. You teach people how to treat you by deciding what you will and won't accept*" Anna Taylor.

Too many of us have the *people pleaser complex*. The need to be a good girl.

As a result, have you ever said yes to something even though it actually depleted what energy you have? It's not about being totally selfish, it's about being *helpful where you can* and want to be helpful but feeling *ok to say no* when you really can't add something else to your day or your week. When you are asked to do something, listen to your gut feeling. If it's a resounding "yes sure I'd love to help you with that" then great. If inside, you're actually feeling "right now that's the last thing I need" *say no.*

And there's a meme I see often on Facebook which says "*the only people who take issue with you having boundaries are the ones who need your boundaries the most.*" It's so true. When you first start to say no to some people, they aren't going to like it. *Stick with it, they'll get used to it.* And you'll have more energy so when you do decide to help out or join in with something, you're doing it without resentment and with *positive energy.*

ACTION: Go back through your diary or calendar for the last month. How many events or activities were on there that frankly you didn't want to do or drained you to do?

Boundaries in the home to get time for yourself: As a parent, getting that time for headspace can be really hard. Raise your hand if you've gone for a wee and not even managed that without being interrupted? Using the advice above on delegation is key to this. But so is identifying something symbolic, so that other family members know that there are times where your need to be left alone is to be respected. As detailed above, in our home the children have learnt that if I'm rowing, they leave me be. We did this by explaining, and reinforcing. And backing each other up in supporting that time out, so if my husband is in, he would remove them or tell them to come to him. Other people, such as a course delegate on my health coach training, used the lighting of her salt lamp to signify that this was Mummy Time. It doesn't matter what the symbol is, but you need to be clear to everyone in the house why this is important. And be consistent in your use of it so they get used to it being a reality.

ACTION: Think about how you would like to take some time out and how you can signal and explain this to your family. Don't be shy at explaining your displeasure if the time you set aside is not respected!

FIND YOUR TRIBE:

- So *who* else is in your team?
- *Who* is there as back up when the kids are sick?
- *Who* is there when actually you just need a couple of hours to yourself?
- *Who* is there to have a moan to?
- *Who* can you cry on when you feel like crap?

- *Who* can you have a giggle with?
- *Who's* there to step in and collect the kids if you're running late?
- *Who* can you run a work or business dilemma past?
- *Who* gets what it's like to be juggling the things you do?

These can be tough questions if when you ask them, you realise you haven't got a name that springs to mind. For many people gone are the days of having friends you've known all your life or extended family around you, these days many of us have moved towns and cities and struggled to build up new friendships. This is where *finding your tribe is part of self-care.*

It has been shown that women naturally seek out support from other women in times of stress.[xxiv] And having a social network is crucial for our physical and mental health. For me, making friends with some of the mums in my kids' classes has been a way of building that tribe, I can share the highs and lows of trying to raise a healthy happy couple of kids.

Joining *The Unique Mumpreneur*, has also added to the tribe I need to help support me professionally. These women also get how sometimes our to do list falls aside as we spend a night up with a sick child, or we feel bad because we had to miss a sports match due to work. They get it because they're paddling a similar boat.

ACTION: If you don't already have some social meet ups in place, task yourself with getting two dates in the diary for the next month where you meet someone you know (or would like to know better) for coffee or a drink just because it's nice to do so. If there's no one you know

locally, your action is to research what groups are around you locally you might like to join or try out.

For practical help, if we don't have some of these people naturally around us then it may be necessary to also build a list of paid support: do you have two names of trusted babysitters you can pay if needed? Do you have a dog walker or pet sitter you trust to step in? Who solves your frozen laptop crisis? Sometimes, just knowing you have a set of people to call, even if you don't need to do it that often can take away the sense of panic.

ACTION: Make a list of all the tasks that you might need help with if you or your partner are away or sick. Write a name or company beside each task as your back up plan.

A Busy Woman's Support Team

	Name	Telephone Number
Plumber		
Heating Engineer		
Electrician		
Mechanic		
Vets		
Pet Sitter		
Babysitter 1		
Babysitter 2		
Dentist		
Doctor		
IT Person		
Cleaner		
Virtual Assistant		

My Team

CHAPTER 5 YOUR WONDERFUL HORMONES AND HOW IT ALL LINKS TOGETHER

Who remembers the cringe-worthy biology lessons about menstruation?

Did anyone tell you about how your body is basically performing a complex ballet dance of hormonal interactions involving multiple organs every day? Did anyone tell you that your menstrual cycle can tell you a heck of a lot about what else is happening in your body? Of course not!

But even more importantly did anyone tell you all the things that can knock this careful synchronised dance off track and how much power we have to influence this? If you are going to feel well, feel energised, cope with life with its ups and downs, you need to understand that how we live on a daily basis has a direct impact on our hormones.

So here's a whistle stop tour of what's going on and why you need to know it.

Let's start with your **LIVER.** Yes, your liver! I bet you thought I was going to start with your ovaries. We will get to those in a bit.

So, most people know that the liver exists to clear toxins. It also helps regulate our blood sugar by storing sugar and releasing it as required, it produces proteins, it helps fight infections, and it produces compounds that help us absorb vitamins, including vitamin D. It regulates cholesterol. It supports our digestive system by producing bile.

But did you know, it also clears and helps regulate hormones, such as adrenaline, thyroid, cortisone and oestrogen? It does this by producing *Sex Hormone Binding Globulin* (SHBG) which attaches to hormones we don't need and helps clear them.

If we overload our liver by eating too much sugar, or live in a constant state of stress (which raises our blood sugar), the insulin our body releases to handle the excess sugar suppresses the SHBG, meaning the liver can't do its job properly and ends up storing up the hormones we don't need.

Where does this leave us? Hormonally-unbalanced. Bloated. Constipated. Grumpy. Irritable. PMT symptoms. Clotty heavy periods. Low libido. Poor sleep. Hot flushes and mood swings in peri-menopause. Low immunity so we catch every bug going. Excess sugar gets laid down as belly fat.

So what overloads our liver?

- Stress
- Lack of sleep
- Sugary food
- Poor diet lacking in nutrients
- Alcohol
- Chemicals we add to our bodies (for example: processed foods, make up, fake tan, hair dye, shampoos, household chemicals such as air fresheners).

The liver really is a *superhero of an organ* and so much of how we live makes it work harder than it needs to. Leaving us out of balance and not feeling our best self. Our liver can be struggling to work at its best way *before any changes show up on blood tests*. In fact, by the time you get blood results that are out of normal range, your liver will have been *struggling and overwhelmed for quite some time*.

Now let's look at **GUT HEALTH**. Many people have now heard of the *gut-brain connection*. How the "*good bacteria*" of our gut link to our mood. 90% of serotonin, the *"happy" hormone*, is synthesised in our gut and reacts with our gut bacteria to regulate its use throughout the body and impact things like gut motility, immune health, bone health and heart health.[xxv]

If we fill ourselves with processed food, too much sugar and not enough veggies, the balance of gut bacteria is off, leading to low mood and contributing to mental health issues such as *depression and anxiety*.

But our *bowels* also help us clear excess hormones. The fibre in our diet helps sweep away the hormones we don't need (especially important in conditions such as *PCOS and endometriosis*). So if we don't eat enough fibre, the job of clearing excess hormones doesn't get done. So we end up out of balance and the liver has to *work harder*.

Poor gut health also means that the gut can be leaky, which means toxins and micro particles of food that should stay in the gut and be cleared with our bowel movements can escape into the rest of our system. This can causes a number of problems:

- more toxins for the liver to clear.

- Raised levels of inflammation in the body and brain that damage so many aspects of our health (think arteries, brain[xxvi], egg[xxvii] and sperm quality) Brain fog is now believed to be a response to inflammation[xxviii],[xxix] Or our body mounts an immune response to the particles it perceives as foreign invaders and we end up with *auto-immune disorders* (such as thyroid issues, lupus etc). Our mitochondrial function, the process of releasing energy from our cells is also affected.

Poor gut health is now tied to conditions such as *Multiple Sclerosis* and *Parkinson's*.[xxx] Gut health is also linked to many skin conditions such as *acne, eczema* and *psoriasis*. The latest research also finds that our gut health has an impact on how well certain medical treatments like *cancer treatments* work[xxxi]. If our gut is in good health, the treatment is more effective.

Our gut is actually the largest part of our *immune system*. If we don't treat it right, we just won't have good health.

For centuries, the ancient Chinese held that our digestive system was at the heart of our good health and had an impact on *clear thinking* and our *whole ability to thrive*.

Modern scientific methods and discoveries are now taking this even further and in a not too distant future, *individualised analysis of our gut microbiome* will lead to tailored treatments to alter our health.

Already, we are learning that specific bacteria play a role in the development of conditions such as diabetes. The research into all this is extremely exciting! But on a day to day level it comes down to what we put into our bodies and how we live our lives.

> *"With autoimmune disease, the power to turn your life around rests not with your doctor, not with a pharmacist, not in a bottle of pills, but in your own hands. That's scary but incredibly empowering."* Dr Terry Wahls, MD

As leading functional medicine doctor, Dr Mark Hyman says *"what you do with your fork impacts everything."*[xxxii]

So what upsets the balance of our gut?

- Stress
- Lack of sleep
- Sugary diet
- Lack of vegetables
- Environmental toxins
- Chemicals sprayed onto vegetables
- Meat and fish raised using growth hormones and significant volumes of antibiotics
- Processed food (especially artificial sweeteners)
- Unhealthy fats
- Alcohol
- Antibiotics
- Other medicines such as the birth control pill[xxxiii] and proton pump inhibitors (omeprazole, lanzoprazole etc), Non Steroidal Anti Inflammatories (such as ibuprofen)

In the chapter on *Nourish Yourself* there will be more information on what you can do about some of these issues, but, for now let's move onto the next key player in keeping us healthy and hormonally balanced:

OUR BRAIN:: Two key parts of the brain, the *hypothalamus* and the *pituitary gland*, work in partnership with the *adrenal glands* that sit on top of our *kidneys* to control our *stress response*. The *hypothalamus* sits at the base of our brain and when asked to by the feedback response from our body, releases a bunch of chemicals, that tells our *pituitary gland* (which sits not far behind the bridge of your nose) to release the *hormones* our *body needs*.

Our pituitary gland releases:

- Thyroid Stimulating Hormone (TSH) involved in healthy thyroid function.
- Luteinising Hormone (LH) which tells our body when to release an egg in ovulation
- Follicle Stimulating Hormone (FSH) which helps our body ripen our eggs ready for release
- ACTH which tells our adrenal glands to release cortisol, the stress hormone.

When we are stressed, we produce *cortisol* from our adrenal glands on our kidneys. This is a normal and healthy thing for us to do, in fact essential for other functions in the body and is actually an *anti-inflammatory*.

Our body then has a feedback loop, that tells our *brain* when it can stop producing *cortisol*, and we return to a balanced state. The problem comes when we live in a *constant state of stress*. *Cortisol* being present for too long actually then goes on to suppress the actions of the *hypothalamus*, namely the production of a chemical called *GnRH* (gonadotropin releasing hormone) which is what tells our pituitary to release all the hormones we need (like LH and FSH) for *reproductive function*.

It also inhibits another feedback loop, that from our *ovaries* (which release *estradiol* (part of *oestrogen)* and *progesterone*) to our *pituitary* and *hypothalamus* .[xxxiv]

I like to think of it as a *survival mechanism*: If we are in a high state of stress the whole time, the last thing our body needs to worry about is being pregnant, as that would place more demands on us than we might cope with, so it *starts to do away with that function*.

Cortisol also causes our blood sugar to rise as it tells our body to release more *sugar* into our system ready to face the danger it thinks we are in. Which as above, messes with our ability to *clear excess hormones*.

When *cortisol* starts interfering with our *reproductive function* it puts us massively out of balance. So whether getting pregnant is something you want to do or not, it is important for our *overall health and wellbeing* in ways that touch every aspect of our lives.

Your *cortisol* production impacts the ability of your *thyroid* to do its job.

If due to *prolonged cortisol production* or other stress responses, our cells lose their ability to be sensitive to *cortisol -* *inflammation* is allowed to take over throughout our entire system. If our *adrenals* go so far as to no longer being able to produce *cortisol* then *systemic inflammation* is what happens.

Being *hormonally out of balance* also impacts on *heart* health, *brain* health, *mental* health, *weight control* and general sense of *feeling on top form*.

Finally your **OVARIES** and their role in *hormonal balance!*

So you can see that your *whole hormonal system* involves more than just the dodgy diagram of *uterus*, *fallopian tubes* and *ovaries* you were shown at school!

The ovaries are where all your eggs are stored. *You are born with all your eggs.* The carefully choreographed dance of *hormonal signalling* described above means each month one (occasionally two) of your eggs are released.

The process of an egg maturing (*folliculogenesis*) can take around one year and what you eat and drink, particularly in the last 190 days (as that is when the follicles begin to respond to their environment) has an impact on how they mature.[xxxv] Your *ovaries* and *uterus* aren't somehow sealed off from what's happening in the rest of your body.

It's been found that if the fluid around the *follicle* which is maturing the *egg* (so what your *egg* is bathed in as it matures prior to release at *ovulation*) contains too much *glucocorticoid* (*cortisol*), the chances of that *egg* resulting in a *pregnancy* are lower. It has also been found (on studies in mice) that different forms of *stress* reduce the *receptivity of the uterine lining* to *implantation of an embryo*. [xxxvi]

Our *ovaries* produce *oestrogen* and *progesterone*.

Progesterone is what helps us *maintain a pregnancy* once *conception* has taken place. As well as being a key hormone in our *reproductive cycle* (and development of *breasts* and *hips*). Toxins from leaky gut can interfere with progesterone production.[xxxvii] Low progesterone is linked to issues with PMS and can lead to a short luteal phase, impacting our ability to become pregnant.

Oestrogen seems to have a role in protecting our *hearts*, which means once our bodies have less of it after *menopause*, unless we are taking excellent care of ourselves, we are more at risk of *heart disease*. *Oestrogen* also supports our bone production, which is why a drop in *oestrogen* after *menopause* puts some *women* at risk of *osteoporosis* (brittle bones).

Oestrogen helps *regulate cervical mucous* (essential for letting sperm in during our fertile window), and keeps our vaginal walls supple and appropriately lubricated. It also helps keep our *skin* looking young and smooth.

Oestrogen is closely linked to the use of *serotonin*. *Serotonin* is both a *hormone* and *neurotransmitter* and is best known for its impact on our mood. It has many functions throughout the body but it's effect on our mood is also tied to the *fluctuation* of our *oestrogen levels* throughout the *menstrual cycle* as many of our cells have both *oestrogen* and *serotonin receptors*.

It's widely believed that the drop in *oestrogen* as we enter *menopause* is linked via *serotonin* to the *mood fluctuations* that hit women at this time. *Oestrogen* also has a role in our sensitivity to *insulin* and in *cholesterol* production.

Maintaining the correct balance of *oestrogen* with progesterone is also important. Additionally our body being able to metabolise (in the liver) and excrete oestrogen is important and producing too many of certain oestrogen bi-products leads to what is known as oestrogen dominance. Oestrogen dominance contributes to issues like endometriosis and fibroids, systemic inflammation, thyroid dysfunction, and in some cases, certain cancers.

So, things that contribute to oestrogen dominance:

- Stress
- Processed foods
- Chemicals and hormones in our water
- Food (meat and fish) raised using growth hormones
- Unhealthy gut bacteria
- Excess weight
- Vitamin deficiencies
- Alcohol
- Chemicals we use in our daily lives (toiletries, household chemicals etc)
- Plastics (especially when heated)

As our ovaries drift into menopause and after, we do still produce some oestrogen, from our adrenal glands. But here's the thing: *it's the same chemical that is the base substance for both cortisol, oestrogen and progesterone.* If we are stressed, the *body prioritises producing cortisol*, so there's less left to make the bit of oestrogen that keeps us from having the worst of the peri-menopausal symptoms[xxxviii]. Or from having a bit of oestrogen to help protect our heart, to stop us gaining that spare tyre of fat on our bellies or stabilise our mood.

This is why doing our best to *reduce stress is crucial to the kind of transition into menopause* that we have. If we are stressed, our oestrogen levels will drop still further.

In fact, in my clinical experience, where some women seem to crash into severe menopausal symptoms including sudden mood crashes that leave them feeling in total despair and even suicidal, when you question them about what was happening in the months leading up to this sudden crash, there is usually some sort of acute or chronic stress. I believe that where someone is teetering on the brink of imbalance, this is enough to tip them into a catastrophic oestrogen loss that produces these major and serious symptoms.

If this all seems massively complicated, which it is (and this is the most user-friendly reduction of it I could come up with and misses out loads of other chemicals and detail!), the takeaway is this:

> Stress messes up your hormones and makes you not only feel awful but damages your body too.

If we constantly over-stress our body (mentally and physically) and add in loads of things that make it have to work harder than it ought, (processed food, chemicals, alcohol, plastics) and don't give it a chance to rest and recuperate (sleep, good hydration , proper nourishment) we knock the delicate balance of how it all works off

**course. This makes us feel and look awful and can lead to
serious health complications long term**.

However, I'm passionate that *more women understand* how
their bodies actually work. Without this understanding being
simply told to eat healthy or being able to make decisions
about whether medication such as HRT or birth control pills are
the way forward, or whether fertility treatment is the path to go
down will be harder to make and they certainly won't be made
from a position of *informed consent*.

For some using these medications will be absolutely the right
decision. For others, lifestyle change will actually be sufficient
to make a massive difference. For some, a combination of
lifestyle change and medication is the correct path.

The reality of the pressures on the current system of healthcare
is such that your GP simply doesn't have the time to go
through your current lifestyle with you or explain how the way
you live impacts your hormones or your general health.

*My mission is to get as many women as possible to understand
that they have the power to make a huge difference to their
own health. And that Putting Yourself First is crucial to this*.

Your mid 30s-40s are really your chance to try and get your
hormonal house in order prior to heading into the peri-
menopause and menopause. The more in balance your body
before you reach this stage, the more chance you have of
avoiding the worst of peri menopausal symptoms. And it
doesn't just affect hormonal health, but studies show how
healthy we are in our 40s has a direct impact on likelihood of

heart disease, diabetes and cognitive health as we get older.[xxxix][xl] This is one of the reasons you really can't wait to put yourself first.

In fact, all of this becomes even more important when we look at how poorly women's health has been prioritised by research and the medical profession over the centuries.[xli] We cannot allow ourselves to rely solely on the research into new medications or conditions to protect us. Chances are they benefit men more than women and chances are you will have to fight harder to be listened to in the first place.[xlii]

Putting yourself first is about trying to maximise your potential to stay well for as long as possible, so you don't need to rely on pharmaceutical treatment in the first place. It's not just about staying alive, but thriving.

LISTENING TO OUR BODIES AND USING OUR CYCLE TO OUR OWN ADVANTAGE

So really, if you think about what you've read above, our bodies are constantly trying to let us know what is wrong and what is right. So many of the annoying or niggling issues we experience are actually *signals from our body* that we are not in balance.

Any woman who has visited a professional acupuncturist will know that we set a lot of store by the signals our body is giving us. Are we inflamed? Are we depleted? Are we consumed by stress and unexpressed emotion? Is our digestive system on fire or out of energy all together?

Our bodies are sometimes quite literally *screaming* at us but in modern times we have been taught to ignore these things and our instincts are dulled as to what is happening.

When it comes to periods, they are really a bit of a secret superpower letting us know what's happening systemically. *Our periods are a reflection of the whole-state of us.*

What goes on in your emotions and the rest of your body is telling us a lot through how you feel before during and after your period. If a person is very well balanced the arrival of their period is without pain, irritability or anxiety, or energy loss. The blood appears in a decent amount, not spotting and threatening to appear for days, the bleed is pain free, doesn't flood, no clots or mucous, lasts about three to five days and when it finishes there's a clean stop, no spotting or bits for another few days.

If you're now saying *"yeah right!"* I hear you. Most of us are some way out of balance, physically and emotionally. Unfortunately *it's now become the norm to be out of balance.* In my acupuncture clinic I often see women for issues around headaches or anxiety and stress. These women are usually surprised when as well as feeling better in themselves their periods also become less problematic.

Below is a handy summary of how a traditionally trained professional acupuncturist (contact the British Acupuncture Council to find one) interprets your period (bear in mind this is a very simplified version and most people are a complex mix) that might help you reflect on where you at overall physically and emotionally.

Note, many of these things come under the description of "normal" according to doctors and gynaecologists. *Normal doesn't necessarily mean optimal* and whilst some of these are not reflective of a disorder and disease in your body, they may not be making life as pleasant as it could be.

Some can be indicative of underlying issues such as fibroids or endometriosis so if you're not sure, always get checked out by a doctor.

Painful cramps just before and at the start of your period	Stuck emotions, especially anger or frustration, stress, lack of physical movement
Big chunky clots	Heat and inflammation in the body, stagnation of blood from keeping emotions locked down for too long
Lots of small clots	Cold in the body, lack of good flow, lack of warming foods
Very dark red/black blood	Stagnation of blood, not enough movement in the body.
Brown blood	Stagnation of blood or not enough energy to expel the last of the old blood
Very light flow	Deficient in nutrients and good blood flow to the uterus to create a good lining
Flooding/heavy flow	Heat/inflammation in the body

Exhausted after your period	Run down and depleted, especially in things like iron rich foods
Irritable/emotional prior to period	Stuck emotions, frustration, anger, not expressing what you want to say
Carb cravings before period	Blood sugar balance not optimal as easily derailed by hormonal shifts, lacking in certain nutrients
No energy prior to the start of period	Stuck energy and emotions, overall run down and depleted.

As you can see words like "stagnation or stuck" come up a lot. This is because the ancient Chinese believed that aside from Invading Pathogens (viruses, bacterial infections, heat or cold exposure etc) *the root of all ill health is the emotions*.

The clue is in the word, eMOTIONs.[xliii] It's normal to have all sorts of different emotions, grief, anger, sadness, fear, joy, excitement etc, but if they don't *flow* through you but get *stuck*, through lack of acknowledgement, inability or lack of opportunity or awareness to express them, they stagnate, almost like rubbish that starts to rot, it gradually affects everything around it, spreading illness and ill health.

In Chinese medicine, different organs are particularly affected by different emotions. For example grief affects the lungs (ever noticed how someone gets cold after cold when they've been bereaved?), worry affects the digestion, anger affects the liver (irritable when you've got repressed anger?) and fear affects the kidneys.

We cannot run from our unresolved emotions. At some point our body finds a way to express them, usually through ill health.

This is where taking time to sit with emotions we feel and let them flow is so important, and why practices such as mindfulness or meditation are so important for health. Mindfulness in particular allows us to just observe what is going on within us without judgement. Sometimes just acknowledging that we have an unresolved emotion is enough to take the pressure off. See the section on relaxation in the chapter Nourish Yourself for more on this.

As women, we have historically had our emotions belittled, ignored and downplayed or ridiculed. Even the word Hysteria (from the Greek word for uterus) has its roots in undermining our emotions as if we are irrational or incapable due to being female.

Look at the number of women who have been repressed, sexually assaulted or exploited, or how as young girls we are taught to be polite and respectable instead of expressing our true thoughts.

Look at how we have to think of all these things just to walk down a street at night. We don't have to look too hard to see how women expressing anger or outrage are deemed as out of control but when a man does it it's just expressing himself or showing his strength through feeling.

And societally, women have a lot to grieve, a lot to be angry about and one hell of a lot of frustration.

It's no wonder at all that periods have become normalised as painful and troublesome as living with stuck emotions has become our norm.

Now we throw into the mix modern life with it's array of harmful chemicals, food that is no longer as nutritious as it once was, lack of time, lots of stress, expectation and pressure and really, we are like powder kegs.

We will go one of two ways, damp and depleted and no energy to light the spark for the powder keg to go off, so we never reach potential and live in a state of exhaustion and sadness, or we explode in a cascade of inflammatory self-destruction, pain, anger and active disease.

Our bodies are often a mix of the two, one part simmering away in pain and disease, the other part too exhausted to change.

But this is where taking the time to Put Yourself First is so important. Taking that time to exercise and move, to relax, to nourish yourself, to acknowledge your achievements and all you've been up against is not a luxury. It's essential for your health.

Not only can you use your period to tell you about what's going on, you can use the whole of your cycle to *your own advantage.*

Each of us experience the menstrual cycle in slightly different ways. The important thing is to learn how different parts of your cycle affect *you personally.* Which days are you low mood?

Which days are you bursting with energy and ideas? Which days are you quieter and more introspective? Which days are you more impulsive? If you start paying attention you'll notice that there are *patterns* to your feelings and energy levels. *Work with them*!

There's no point in trying to plan marketing and new ideas for your business or job when you are on a day that you are naturally low mood and more reflective. That day would be better spent catching up on admin tasks! It's definitely not a good idea to make big decisions on days you have low optimism.

Have you noticed how around ovulation you are either energetic or really grumpy? Again, a reflection of how smoothly transitions from one stage to another (from follicular phase to ovulation to luteal phase) are moving for you.

Personally speaking, I've noticed that often just before ovulation I'm convinced my practice is failing, nothing is working and I'm generally a bit low (yes i am also out of balance, I am a work in progress like all of us are!). Now I know that this can happen (not every month as the months I've got everything else more in balance this is less obvious) I don't worry about it. I tell myself just to ignore any such worries and think about them in a few days.

And I use it as a barometer of where I'm at in my self-care.

If I'm particularly low at that time, I know I've not been resting or relaxing and de-stressing enough. Just after a period or a couple of days after ovulation I'm on fire! Energetic, positive, I can do it all! This is a wonderful time to crack on with new projects, planning ideas, writing new blog posts, signing up to events that challenge me out my comfort zone. If you're exhausted in this phase, chances are you are *run down* and *depleted in essential nutrients*. Then, as my period comes, it's a time for lazy baths, reading novels, watching back to back Outlander episodes and generally *nurturing* myself.

Our hormones are not doing the same thing every day, so why do we expect our bodies and minds to function each day as if this cycle were not happening?

The whole of work-culture is set up around the less dramatic fluctuation of the male body. There are a few more forward-thinking businesses, who now acknowledge that the female menstrual cycle directly affects how their employees function and offer them greater flexibility around their work during their period. But most women cannot wait for the world of work to catch up to this, and will have to resort to working around this themselves.

For those of us raising daughters, this fluctuation of feeling more inspired and brave can also translate into *riskier adolescent behaviour* depending on where in their cycle the girls are at! (Week 2 of the follicular phase)[xliv]. Let us educate our girls to understand their cyclical fluctuations so they can be more self-aware and more *empowered* in their own bodies!

Broadly speaking, our menstrual cycle is in four parts: our period, the follicular phase where we are preparing an egg to be ovulated, ovulation, and the luteal phase where our body is waiting to see if conception has happened and an embryo implanted.

Traditionally, our period is a time for rest and nurturing ourselves.

The first day of our period is known as day 1. The follicular phase is when we blossom, feel energetic and as we enter our fertile window roughly 4 days before we ovulate, we can become our most attractive (think bright eyes, attractive pheromones, slightly more rounded hips and breasts, clear stretchy egg-white cervical mucous that allows sperm to enter the uterus).

For the record, ovulation is only at day 14 in around 10% of 28 day cycles[xlv]. For some women ovulation is anywhere from day 10 to 22. (If you have PCOS, it can be not at all or only every few months).

After ovulation, our progesterone levels rise to help support a potential pregnancy and this brings greater energy, until our body realises we aren't pregnant, hormone levels start to drop and a few days later our period begins. This phase, known as the luteal phase is generally10-14 days long. Any longer or shorter and you are looking at imbalances that need checking out.

Or, if you are exhausted and in pain throughout your cycle, you need to be checked.

It's at these points of fluctuation, transition to period, transition to ovulation, transition towards our period, that our most extreme *fluctuations in mood* can occur. And as per the last chapter, all of these fluctuations and transitions are affected *by stress, sugar, alcohol, sleep and nutrition*.

If you want to learn about tracking your cycle in more depth then check out the book Period Power by Maisie Hill. She goes deep into each phase of the menstrual cycle, calling the four-phases Winter, Spring, Summer and Autumn. She also explores in detail the transition into puberty and menopause, the effects of different methods of hormonal birth control, emotions and issues around hormonal imbalance.[xlvi]

Learning what is normal for you also helps you spot any changes that could be signs of disease or ill-health. *As a rule of thumb, anything that is not normal for you needs checking*.

Your vaginal discharge is another great tool for telling you how things are going. It is normal to have different types of discharge throughout your cycle. From just a small amount, to what seems like copious quantities, from creamy coloured, to clear and stretchy, to thicker and cloudy, it's all part of being a woman. And it just wasn't talked about when we were growing up.

If it changes, to green, to smelling offensive, to itchy, something is not right and needs checking. Burning sensations, soreness, blood when it's not your period or after sex, again, all need checking by the doctor.

All women should read Taking Charge of Your Own Fertility by Toni Weschler.[xlvii] It's not just essential reading if you want to become pregnant, it's essential reading for understanding your own body and helping yourself stay healthy.

As well as being taught about periods, young girls should be taught about the cyclical changes of their discharge so they are more aware and more in control of where they are at with their health, their hormones, their fertility, their choices. They also need to be taught about what is normal with their external genitalia and their sexual health, without being ashamed. Another good book for this is The Gynae Geek.[xlviii]

As we head into the peri-menopause, acknowledging what is happening in your body becomes even more important. What changes are taking place? Are your moods more extreme? Are your periods shorter and closer together?

Again, *your body is a barometer* of how smoothly changes are happening. If you are in balance, we transition smoothly from the fertile period of our life to the non-fertile but no less valuable post-menopausal phase. The more you struggle with this phase of your life, the more likely it is that you are in real need of *radical self-care*.

From the ancient Chinese perspective, our lives are made up of movement from yin (nurturing, growing, thoughtful, cooling) to yang (movement, energetic, warming). We flow from one into the other, in our monthly cycles, from day to night, from childhood to puberty, from fertile years to menopause. *It's where there is no smooth flow that ill health or distress occurs.*

CHAPTER 6 SLEEP YOURSELF HEALTHY

If you want to thrive, and indeed, survive, it's essential to Put Yourself First when it comes to sleep.

Sleep really is up there as a cornerstone of our health. There's a reason that sleep deprivation is used as a form of torture by nasty regimes around the world. You can only go a few days without sleep before you sink into delirium, hallucination and even psychotic episodes.

Now, while the vast majority of us have never experienced sustained continual sleep deprivation, it's estimated 74% of us get by on less than 7 hours sleep a night and over a third of us getting by on less than 5-6 hours a night [xlix]. And 12% of us on less than five hours. And guess what? Women tend to get less sleep than men! So most of us are suffering chronic sleep deprivation, where we are not getting the optimum hours or quality of sleep for *good physical and mental health.*

Being chronically short on sleep has the following effects on our bodies:

- Weight gain
- Hormonal imbalance
- Low mood and greater risk of depression and anxiety
- Increased risk of illness from inflammatory conditions: diabetes, heart disease, stroke, acid reflux
- Increased risk of cognitive decline as we age
- Greater risk of accidents (a sleep deprived driver can be as dangerous as a drunk driver).

- Lower motivation to make healthy choices (smoking, drinking alcohol, picking sugary fatty foods)
- Your immune system and ability to heal is compromised so you get sick all the time and take longer to recover.

So you can see that without working on your sleep, all the other chapters of this book are kind of redundant. Yes, the advice in the other chapters feeds into creating good sleep, but your chances of implementing any of it are somewhat lower if you don't *follow this chapter first.*

So what is 'enough' sleep?

For the average person *7-9 hours sleep is optimal.* Yes, we've all heard the stories of famous politicians who only slept 3-4 hours a night and achieved great things. Delve a little deeper and most of them ended their days with problems like Alzheimer's or stroke.

And yes, there is a tiny percentage of people who have a genetic variation that means they can get by on much less sleep than the rest of us. But it's probably fair to assume you're not one of those people. So assume you're a mere average mortal being who needs *7-8 hours a night.*

So ask yourself the following question: do you actually spend at least 8 hours physically in bed every night? It's normal during a night time to move through different phases of sleep, from light to deep to REM dream sleep.

We need to spend time in each of these phases for our brains and bodies to make the necessary repairs. It's also normal for it to take a certain amount of time to drop off (approximately 15-20 mins) and to have episodes that we may or may not be aware of where we rouse in the night and are technically not in sleep state.

The average time to be classed as "awake" during the night for women late 30s to mid 40s is 10-20%. So to actually get 7 hours sleep, realistically you actually need to be in bed for 8 whole hours.

ACTION: Keep a note over the next week of the time you lie down and switch out your light, and the time you wake up in the morning. How many hours are you actually in bed for every night?

It's not just quantity, but *quality*!

Ever technically had a long sleep but woken up feeling sluggish or like you've had much less sleep than you had? Or ever had not so many hours but woken up feeling not too bad?

Chances are if you're feeling tired after enough sleep you've not had enough time in a *deep sleep state*, or too much in dream state or light sleep. Or if you were short on sleep but felt good, you might have had optimal time in *deep sleep*, but skipped out on some light sleep.

The beauty of some of the modern wearable health trackers is that you can find out what's going on for you. On a personal level I've noticed that if I get about 1 hour 20 to 1 hour 30 in the deep sleep zone I feel energised and able to think clearly. If I get less than this it takes me longer to get going and I don't feel that I function at full throttle. If I get less than an hour deep sleep, then it's a survival mode kind of day.

You don't need to rush out and buy such a device, and for some people wearing them and looking at numbers and statistics stresses them out more than it empowers them, the point to take away is, quality of sleep is also hugely important.

The latest research tells us that when we enter a deep sleep brain, our brain is flooded and effectively washed in cerebro-spinal fluid, clearing away toxins. So if we don't enter deep sleep, we don't get that brain refresh, which long-term has implications for conditions such as Alzheimers.[1]

Things that affect the *quality of our sleep* are:

- Stress levels (the stress hormone cortisol can interfere with the sleep hormone melatonin)
- Blood sugar imbalances (waking up repeatedly around 4:30am can be a sign of this)
- Wired brain (brains process all we have seen during the day while we sleep, exposure to lots of screen time especially in the evening over stimulates the brain so it's still firing on all cylinders instead of resting)
- Caffeine: it's a stimulant and takes 12 hours to clear our systems, so that afternoon tea or coffee could be affecting your sleep
- Alcohol: also a stimulant and actually the last thing we should use to unwind in the evening
- Room temperature: too hot or too cold you'll toss and turn. 16-18 degrees Celsius is optimal.

- Hydration levels: many don't drink enough in the day. Being mildly dehydrated can cause us to rouse from deep sleep
- Restless partners : this is so real! Snoring too. It's not just yourself needs to be worked on sometimes!
- Children: they cry, they wake us, but also when small we sleep with a listening ear. Or they just end up in our beds.
- Pregnancy: we need to pee, we're uncomfortable, everything aches
- Hormonal cycle: this can affect sleep quality and body temperature
- Bladder problems: if you're struggling with irritable bladder or continence issues, this will have you up at night.
- Pain: physical ailments that mean we can't get comfy will stop us sleeping
- Depression or anxiety: disturbed sleep can be a sign and a cause of mental health problems
- Worries: fretting about things that are worrying us, means it can take longer to drop off and when we enter lighter sleep states we are more likely to wake if our brain is whirring
- Vitamin and mineral deficiencies : being deficient in certain vitamins and minerals such as Vitamin D, the B vitamins, iron and magnesium can make it harder to sleep well.
- Exercise: too little, too much or at the wrong time of day for us means less than optimal sleep
- Eating late: simply, our digestive system should be resting at night so all our resources go into repair mode. If your body is still busy trying to digest food at the least

efficient time of the day to do so it's not going to switch into rest and repair mode so easily.

- Light: too many devices with charging lights, street lights, alarm clocks all stop it from being dark about to sleep well. Exposure to the wrong types of light (bright white LED) from bulbs or laptops/phones/tablets (blue light) also makes our brain think it's still daytime.

That's quite a list! So it's no wonder really many of us struggle to feel rested. Trying to work out which of those are affecting us personally isn't always easy.

ACTION: Over a week, make a note of how you feel after your sleep, whether it's energised or exhausted, make a note of what you ate and drank the day before, what you did in the hours leading up to bedtime, where you were in your menstrual cycle, what was going on for you with stress etc. You'll soon start to learn what affects your own sleep.

So what can we do to actually get enough sleep?

1. Top of the list has to be *go to bed on time* (as in be in bed lights out 8 hours before you need to be up)!!! And for many women this is just not as easy as that sounds.

How many of us get to the time we want to go to bed, go to lock up or take a cup into the kitchen and end up tidying up? Or your child's swim kit isn't in a bag in the hallway ready to go, or the cat bowl needs topping up? So you do all that and although you started to go to bed on time, by the time you actually get into bed it's at least an hour later? How many of your partners declare they are going to bed, stand up from the sofa, walk upstairs, climb into bed and go to sleep? Familiar? It's a classic case of women putting themselves behind the needs of everyone else in the family.

But there is a way to change this. It takes time and effort to implement but is certainly possible and really quite liberating so read on!

The bedtime routine for the household actually needs to start the moment everyone comes home through the door from school or work. It's the responsibility of every single person to ensure their dirty lunch boxes or gym kit are taken to the dishwasher or washing machine before they start playing or watching telly. *Any child capable of going to school is capable of doing this*.

Bedtime for the children starts by helping younger ones and making older ones ensure all uniform or kit for the following day is packed into the relevant bags or laid out ready. Once the younger kids are dispatched to bed, yourself or your partner or older children can make the lunch boxes and do the dishwasher. *Nobody sits down until the house is ready for the next day.*

Sounds strict? Think you'll face a rebellion? You probably will, but please jump to the chapter on **DELEGATION** for tips on how to do this. *But persevere*. It will be tough creating this new routine. Your household needs to work as a team. If they want a mum or partner who is fun and cheery and positive, *they need a mum who is rested*.

That first evening you manage to sit down to watch something you want to watch on telly and know everything is done and you can just go straight to bed when you are ready is liberating and you'll wonder why you didn't do it years ago.

ACTION: Sit down with a pen and paper and make a list of everything that needs to happen each evening so the household is ready for the following day. Work out by age appropriateness, who can do what and when. Then have a discussion with your partner about the changes that need to happen and why. And present the changes to the kids. Implement the new routine.

2. *Work on your sleeping environment*: is it dark enough? Do you need thicker curtains or a sleep mask? Are there clocks with bright screens or chargers with flashing lights? Turn them around or move them elsewhere. Are the lamps beside your bed too bright? Can they be changed to a more yellow light bulb? Have you switched all your devices into orange light mode at sunset to sunrise?

ACTION: Carry out a little survey of your room. Make any required changes.

3. *Put any devices with screens across the room or preferably in another room*. This will help with the urge to scroll whilst lying in bed. You'll find it hard to do this at first if lying in bed scrolling is something you normally do, so have something else at hand, a book, crossword, sudoku, audio book, or even, just talk or make love with your other half!

ACTION: Consider what you can use to replace scrolling and ensure it's beside your bed, whilst your phone is as far away as possible.

4. *Consider your bedding*: does one of you get too hot and the other too cold? Does your other half toss and turn and steal the duvet each time? Consider separate duvets that suit each of your needs, and then use a bedspread or throw over the top when the bed is made to keep it looking nice.

5. *Practice gratitude or breathing exercises* once in bed to get your body into a state of relaxation. Sounds corny, but lying there thinking of all the things/people you are grateful for can really help induce a feeling of wellbeing and calm that helps us drift off.

ACTION: Lie in bed and think of at least five things for which you are grateful.

6. *Look at the list above* about the causes of poor quality sleep: Are there any reasons that stand out to you? Which of them do you need to work on? Do you need to seek medical help or see a nutritionist? Do you need guidance on helping your child with their sleep routine? Does your partner need to seek any help for their issues which are disturbing you?

7. *Replace evening stimulants such as caffeine and alcohol* with non-sugary drinks like chamomile tea or other calming herbal teas. No one's saying never drink again, but give this a go for a good while and see the difference it makes.

ACTION: Check you've got herbal teas in the house or add them to the shopping list

8. If you don't do some form of *daily exercise*, try and incorporate an outdoor walk into your daily life. In an ideal world it would be in the morning. Being exposed to daylight helps regulate melatonin (the sleep hormone) and a walk in nature helps relax us and tire our bodies physically not just mentally.

ACTION: Look at your daily routine. How can you get into daylight each day?

9. If you do *regular exercise*, consider whether your sleep is better or worse depending on the time of day you are doing it? Is it worse if you do an evening work out? You might need to switch up your routine to work out first thing, and do something calming like yoga or meditation in the evening.

ACTION: Keep a note of when you exercise and see if there's any pattern between when you exercise and your sleep.

10. *Try not to eat late where possible*, but when it can't be helped, don't have a meal full of carbs or sugar, try more sleep promoting foods such as almonds (they contain melatonin and magnesium), turkey (contains tryptophan which helps produce melatonin), kiwi (contains serotonin and antioxidants) or oily fish (contains vitamin D, omega 3 and fatty acid). See the chapter on Nourish Yourself for more advice on eating for health.

11. *Work on stress reduction*: easier said than done but see the chapters on delegation and Nourish Yourself. But good at bedtime is a relaxing bath with Epsom salts (the magnesium in them helps relax us). Have regular acupuncture or massages and use meditation and mindfulness apps once a day.

CHAPTER 7 NOURISH YOURSELF: What to put in and what to take out

This chapter aims to unravel some of the mysteries around what we can do on a real and daily level to stay well in our busy lives. The aim has to be to prevent ill health from occurring in the first place.

From what to eat, to diet, exercise and how to de-stress, I'm going to share with you ideas for you to take away and then apply to your own life. There's *no magic bullet*, no one thing that if you do you'll live a sun-filled shiny joyful existence. But cumulatively, you'll feel better and more in control of your own health.

Use this chapter as a springboard to learn more about what you can do and *how much power you have over your own life and health*. Each thing I suggest is the subject of many more in-depth books so feel free to take a deeper dive into each suggestion.

You don't have to dive into each of these things in one go if that doesn't work for you. Pick the one you feel most able to tackle and work on it until it becomes part of your daily life. Then move on to the next one.

You will notice that a significant chunk of what is written is about what you eat and drink. In Chinese medicine, *food is the first and most powerful medicine*. Think about it. Each bite you take is made up of a complex set of cells, that interact with our own cells and bacteria, to produce an effect that is either helping us, or harming us. We all eat. Three or more times a day. It's the biggest thing we all do.

In terms of putting yourself first, aside from sleep, *eating well is one of the greatest things we can do for ourselves.* It is our most powerful weapon in the quest to not just survive, but thrive.

If you are stuck with knowing where to start on how to tackle each of the suggestions below, consider working with a health coach who can help you unravel where you are at with each of them, what's happening for you and help you come up with ways you can take steps to better health that fit with your life and goals.

EAT MORE VEG

If we look at the Blue Zones around the world and the studies into the diets of those who live not just the longest, but *stay well the longest,* here are the things they have in common[li]:

    i.   They are mostly plant based
    ii.   They are local and seasonal
    iii.   They aren't processed.

We all know we are meant to eat more vegetables. The UK government recommends a minimum of 5 portions (400g) a day. This is a MINIMUM and not the ultimate goal. And yet only 29% of adults and 18% of children manage this on a regular basis[lii][liii].

In actual fact, for health, it's recommended we eat ten, yes TEN portions a day. It's not as scary as it sounds if you think a portion is 80g, so three heaped tablespoons of peas is a portion. The study showed you can reduce your risk of heart disease (the biggest killer of women) by 28% and premature death by 31% if you eat ten portions a day.[liv]

Variety is also key. The health of your gut bacteria as discussed in a previous chapter, is essential for supporting your immune system, healthy cell function, keeping inflammation at bay, keeping your brain and body healthy and helping with hormonal balance. Plant based food also contains many antioxidants, vitamins, fibre and other goodness essential for our cellular and brain function.

It's not enough to eat the same few vegetables over and over to achieve a good diversity of gut bacteria. The American Gut Project found that those who eat *30 different varieties* of plant a week had a greater diversity of gut bacteria than those eating ten.[lv]

For the purposes of "plant" this also means beans, nuts, lentils, seeds; anything that came from a plant. There are hundreds of variety of edible plants out there, we have just got in a rut at what we think we can eat.

Including fermented foods in your diet is also really helpful for encouraging good diversity of gut bacteria. Think pickles, sauerkraut, even some olives.

Take a look at your local farm shop and count the variety of veg. Go for the *colours of the rainbow* to help with variety. Dark red veg like beetroot, green leafy stuff like kale and chard, orange squashes, yellow peppers, white leeks, cauliflower. Now have a look at garden plants you don't think of as food, like dandelion leaves, nettles or marigolds. It's there all around us, if we know how to look.

You might be thinking this sounds like an impossible task. So here are some handy hints.

Breakfast: if you get a couple of portions in at breakfast you'll likely manage your ten portions that day.

- Ways to do this are:
- Wilted spinach alongside an omelette, with chopped tomato.
- Mixed berries on top of porridge
- Avocado with your egg,
- Frittata with a variety of veg
- Mushrooms alongside your egg
- A banana with a handful of nuts
- Poached pears on your porridge
- Overnight oats with berries, nuts and seeds (chia and flaxeed are good in porridge)

If speed is of the essence, a smoothie is super easy: large handful of chard or spinach, chunk of carrot or beetroot an apple, kiwi or blueberries, some water. If you want more of a thick shake add some oats or some natural yoghurt. Make it up as you go along! Experiment. As long as the bulk of what's in it is veg not fruit you won't need to worry so much about spiking your blood sugar.

Remember that the idea of breakfast being only cereals and toast is an invention of the food industry to sell their products. Around the world people eat leftovers from dinner, noodles and veg, rice and veg and many other varieties of things we wouldn't think of as breakfast. *There are no actual rules as to what breakfast should be.*

So get *creative*.

Lunch:

- Homemade vegetable soup, preferably chunky. Make a big batch and freeze it in portions sizes.
- A salad mixed with a variety of leaves, tomatoes, avocados, radishes, green beans, chickpeas carrots...anything goes! You can easily get 3-4 portions in this way, and really add in variety. Add in a protein of your choice, cheese, chicken, fish, hummus, kidney beans etc. Some oat cakes, or brown rice, lentils, quinoa, to accompany it. A sprinkle of pumpkin seeds on top.
- Last night's leftovers and a piece of fruit.
- Again, look for inspiration and invest in some decent lunch boxes so you can bring warm food, or keep stuff cold. You'll also save a lot of money not spending £3-10 a day on a lunch that's not really nourishing you.

Dinner:

Aside from having stir fry or steamed veg on your plate, you can add it in to so many dishes. A family-friendly way to get things like kale or beetroot in is to hide it in the sauce that makes your shepherd's pie or Spag Bol. Blitz it in and as it simmers down, nobody will notice. Add in sweet potato or butternut squash into the mash. My record is 10 different types of veg hidden in a shepherds pie! You can leave the more kid-friendly stuff in chunks, like carrots and peas, but hide the stuff that might lead to protests.

Again, make big dishes and freeze it in portions. You can add some lentils into the mince and help keep the cost down by making a smaller portion of high quality mince go further. For plant based inspiration check out *Deliciously Ella* or the *Riverford* cookbooks. Get creative. Once this becomes your new normal it will become easier.

Eating seasonally is also helpful for the body. Having a plate of raw salad in the depths of winter will overly challenge your digestive system more than a warming vegetable soup. Adding herbs and spices will not only add flavour and help you avoid processed sauces, but many have medicinal properties that will enhance digestion and well-being.

If you don't eat many veg already, then *pick one meal to focus on getting more veg into* first, and build your repertoire of recipes gradually or you may find it's just too much to bother with and give up.

If you aren't vegetarian, see if you can introduce more meals into your week that are entirely plant based. *We just don't need to eat as much meat as we do*, for health, and for the planet. And if you are vegetarian, see how many meals you are relying on meat-style products and see if you can change that balance.

One Week Veg Challenge Planner

	Monday	Tuesday	Wednesday	Thursday	Friday	Saturday	Sunday
Breakfast	Veg 1: Veg 2: Veg 3:	Veg 1: Veg 2: Veg 3:	Veg 1: Veg 2: Veg 3:	Veg 1: Veg 2: Veg 3:	Veg 1: Veg 2: Veg 3:	Veg 1: Veg 2: Veg 3:	Veg 1: Veg 2: Veg 3:
Lunch	Veg 1: Veg 2: Veg 3:	Veg 1: Veg 2: Veg 3:	Veg 1: Veg 2: Veg 3:	Veg 1: Veg 2: Veg 3:	Veg 1: Veg 2: Veg 3:	Veg 1: Veg 2: Veg 3:	Veg 1: Veg 2: Veg 3:
Dinner	Veg 1: Veg 2: Veg 3:	Veg 1: Veg 2: Veg 3:	Veg 1: Veg 2: Veg 3:	Veg 1: Veg 2: Veg 3:	Veg 1: Veg 2: Veg 3:	Veg 1: Veg 2: Veg 3:	Veg 1: Veg 2: Veg 3:
Total Daily Veg							

ACTION: Have a look at the veg challenge chart. Fill it in in one colour or pencil for the number of portions of veg you get in over the next week. See where you can work on adding more. Fill it in a different colour or rub it out and fill it in again as you challenge yourself each week to add more veg. Add in any fruits you have in the space at the top of each box, but keep your focus on the veg

ACTION: Remember, the key to a healthy habit is making it the easiest thing to do. Reflect on how getting veg into your diet can become the easy thing. Is it having a veg box delivered? Is it growing your own (a planter of kale is the easiest thing to grow!), is it meal prep?

CUT OUT PROCESSED FOOD AND CHEMICALS

One of our major health problems is that much of what we eat isn't really food.

The well-known functional medicine doctor, Dr Mark Hyman calls most of what makes up the SAD diet (Standard American Diet which is pretty similar to what many eat in the UK), *frankenfood*. In other words, a cocktail of chemicals and additives that have no place in our bodies.

Consuming 400 calories on a portion of nuggets or large fries is not the same as 400 calories from a bowl of kale, salmon, chickpeas, greens, almonds.

So many of us now are deplete in essential vitamins and nutrients, but are overeating in terms of calories. But for the average busy person knowing what to buy and eat is confusing and complex. Do start reading labels to see the chemical cocktail that goes into products. The basic rule of thumb should be this, if it's not a dried food, like rice, if it can last months in your cupboard, it's got added stuff in it. Try and eat as little of this as possible.

Cooking from scratch with *real ingredients* is the best way. For many, time and cooking skills are the real issue here. But thanks to the internet, there are videos to watch to teach you the basics. Learn a few key recipes and go from there.

It's not about never having another take-away, it's about making sure that at least 80% of the time what you eat is actually benefiting not harming your body.

Get into batch cooking, plan meals, freeze them, use a slow-cooker to chuck stuff in and leave on all day. Nobody is saying go home today and chuck the contents of your cupboards out, but do start thinking about what you are actually putting on your fork and start the transition to *eating for health not just fuel*. When you eat a meal or a snack ask yourself:

Is this *nourishing* me or *harming* me?

ACTION: How many dishes can you cook from scratch (including the sauces in it)? Challenge yourself to learn one new dish a month that you can cook from start to finish and freeze in portions. Within 6 months you'll have 6 go-to dishes that you can cook up at a weekend into maybe two sets of meals for everyone.

ACTION: Remember, the key to healthy habit change is making it the easiest thing to do, not the hardest. Identify some easy and quick meals that can be put together in less than fifteen minutes prep but contain real ingredients. Make sure you have some of the basics in.

And go for *quality over quantity*. This is especially important when it comes to meat and fish products. It's not just about the harmful chemicals added in the growing process. But, a cow or chicken, or fish, fed on a diet that is natural to it, will contain very different levels of nutrients and types of fats to one which has been fed on grains and antibiotics and other chemicals.

I would rather use half the amount of meat in a dish, but have meat that contains more nutrients and fewer chemicals, than more but lower quality. And having less gives a higher likelihood of adding more veg and plant based products into the dish.

For those who are vegetarian or vegan, please take care on some of the meat substitute products. Many of them are full of unhealthy oils and chemicals.

As for your veg, in a perfect world, like your meat or dairy, it would be organic. Not everyone can stretch to this, so ensure at the very least you wash your veg to remove as much of any chemical residue that you can. *It's still better to get more veg into you whether it's organic or not.*

Some fruits and veg are known to be worst affected by chemicals than others, so if you can prioritise these for being organic it would be a good idea. With thanks to the Pesticide Action Network UK for this list of fruit and veg harbouring the greatest cocktails of chemicals:

Grapefruit, orange, lemons, limes, strawberries, pears, grapes, cherries, peaches, parsnips, asparagus, apples and apricots.

Those non-organic fruit and veg containing the least chemical residues:

Beetroot, corn on cob, mushrooms, figs, rhubarb, swede, turnip, onions, avocado, cauliflower, radish, sweet potato, broad beans, leeks, pumpkins and squash.

BALANCE YOUR BLOOD SUGAR:

From everything you've read in the previous chapters, you will by now realise that keeping your blood sugar steady is up there on the list of self-care and hormonal balance. You now understand how sugar impacts on your hormones and the cascade effect of inflammation and ill-health it brings.

You don't have to be as far along the blood sugar imbalance path and be Type 2 diabetic to have issues with this, but that's where we can end up. *Our bodies can be warning us for years in advance that we are on the wrong path.*

The post lunch slump, the mid-afternoon craving for sugar, getting hangry if you leave it too long to eat, not wanting breakfast, rough skin, belly fat, all signs you might be out of balance.

If you are maxing out on the veg and avoiding chemicals and processed food as above, you have already made some big leaps towards better blood sugar balance.

But here are some more steps you can take:

1. Swap high glycaemic (foods that convert to sugar quickly in your body) carbs to low glycaemic. Essentially, as well as limiting cake, chocolate, biscuits etc, this means getting rid of anything white: White bread, white pasta, potatoes in some forms, white rice, couscous. The reason these things turn to sugar so fast, is they've been refined down until they are high in starch and not in protein and fibre. Swap it for things less refined, like pasta made from spelt flour, brown basmati rice, bulgar wheat, lentils, sweet potato, quinoa.

2. Limit your portion of rice/pasta/potato/bread: this shouldn't really take up more than a quarter of your plate. Have boiled new potatoes instead of mash or baked. The other quarter is your protein, the remaining half is veg.

3. Always have some proteins or fats with your carbs, as it slows down how fast it metabolises into sugar in your. blood. So, if you really want toast, have a super seedy slice, with a pure nut butter (one where it's just the nuts whizzed up, not with added oils and sugar), or have it with mackerel, or an egg. Plus veg.

4. In terms of fats, you want to go for the kind that help lower inflammation in the body such as those from: oily fish, nuts, seeds, avocado. A handful of nuts a day is associated with many health benefits. And will help stop you snacking on less nutritious items!

5. Watch *WHEN* you eat. Our bodies are governed by a body clock of processes that are deeply wired within us. For millennia the Chinese have taught that different organ systems of the body have times of the day at which they are at peak function. Turns out that's another thing they were right about.

    Recent research into our circadian rhythms show that we are pre-set for certain functions to be optimised at certain times. Even down to when we lay down new muscle tissue after exercise.

Having access to food and eating at all hours of the day and night is not helpful to the many different repair cycles that need to take place. It takes hours for our digestive system to finish processing the last of what we've eaten, before the body essential goes into repair and restore mode whilst we are sleeping.

If we can't go into repair and restore because you have eaten late, all sorts of processes, including metabolic processes to do with blood sugar are affected.[lvi] A fun fact is that if allowed, your body will *repair 10% of your stomach lining each night*, which helps prevent things like acid indigestion and heartburn.[lvii]

Ideally, there should be a *twelve hour window* between the last thing you eat and drink (apart from clear liquids like water or herbal tea) and your first. So if you finish your evening meal by 7pm, no snacking, and breakfast at 7, you will be helping with weight loss, blood sugar and hormone balance, sleep quality and energy levels.

Keeping this 12 hour gap is a very light version of intermittent fasting and is shown to be beneficial for many of our bodily functions.[lviii] The latest research shows that those who eat all their food within a *10 hour window* experienced weight loss, lower blood pressure and more stable insulin levels.[lix]

For those who are already diabetic or on medication that needs to be taken in the evening with food, do check with your doctor before doing this.

ACTION: Look at your daily schedule, on most days, to get a 12 hour gap, what time would work best to have breakfast and dinner? Aim to eat nothing after your evening meal. Might be tough the first few nights but have warm herbal teas so you feel you are having something and within a week you will stop missing the evening snack.

6. Manage stress: when we are stressed the cortisol we produce also encourages us to release sugar into our blood stream so it's ready to be used by our muscles to run away from the sabre tooth tiger, or in more modern times, our never ending to do list, financial worries and work worries. This feeds into the vicious cycle of inflammation, insulin resistance and hormonal imbalance. It can mean that even if you are eating super blood-sugar balancing foods, your sugars can still end up higher than they ought to be. See below for tips on managing stress.

THE GLUTEN QUESTION:

Gluten, the sticky proteins contained within wheat and other grains, has become a topic for hot debate with many criticising the current trends of people saying they are intolerant to gluten. As with all things there is an element of truth in both sides.

For sure, those who suffer from the serious illness, coeliac disease; where eating gluten provokes a severe immune response absolutely must avoid gluten to the max. It's estimated 1% of the population have coeliac disease, of which's 30% are undiagnosed (coeliac.org.uk). So there are definitely some people for whom gluten is causing serious harm and yet they don't realise it. Some argue that unless you have coeliac disease, eating gluten is not a problem. And yet many report they feel better off of it.

However, there are those who argue that gluten causes an inflammatory gut response in healthy people.[ix] And whilst not enough to provoke the severe symptoms that someone with coeliac experiences, if we consider the importance of gut health to our systemic inflammation, brain health, mental health, hormonal balance etc the argument for not consuming gluten carries weight.

Meanwhile, other evidence points to gluten avoidance being beneficial for patients with gastro-intestinal symptoms such as IBS, but for other issues the evidence is still lacking[xi]. Though, as we know, lack of evidence is not the same as being proven not to be beneficial for others. Certainly many of those who follow a version of the paleo diet under the Wahls Protocol for addressing symptoms around Multiple Sclerosis are strong advocates for avoiding gluten when trying to reset gut and brain health. [xii]

There is also a growing argument that those with thyroid issues should avoid gluten, as if the gut is leaky, the micro-particles of gluten that can escape the gut and provoke an inflammatory response look similarly to your thyroid cells, and thus the body is more likely to attack its own thyroid cells.[xiii]

The problem when discussing gluten is that as a substance, it's made up of more than one protein, and people can react to one aspect of it, and not others. For sure, we now eat more gluten than every before. It's in more than just bread, it's in many processed products, even in some chocolates and some cosmetics.

People can end up having it with every meal: toast for breakfast, sandwich at lunch, pasta for dinner. And in many cases, it comes with added chemicals used to ensure longevity on the shelf. The bread making process isn't what it was in our granny's time, and the high-yield commercial wheat crops are stronger in gluten than the flour that used to be produced.

The simplest way to find out if gluten is affecting you is to cut it out for a couple of months or so, see how you feel and then how you feel if you reintroduce it.

But please don't fall into the trap of substituting it with highly processed gluten-free products made with things like rice and potato flour that will massively spike your blood sugars!

If that's too difficult, then look at reducing the amount you eat by making your diet more varied and non-processed. Switch to artisan sour-dough bread, where the fermentation process has reduced the amount of gluten in the loaf.

However, if you feel gluten is part of your problem, it's even more important to address the other aspects of your diet and lifestyle that contribute to the inflammation in your body. For many people, gluten is just one part of a much greater problem of high sugar, highly processed food, high stress, no exercise, not enough sleep, all round imbalance.

DRINK:

It's well known that we are approximately 60% water. So it's crucial to stay well hydrated. You can tell if you are well hydrated by looking at your pee. It should be clear, and pale, kind of like water with a hint of yellow (although certain medications and vitamins can change this). For most people, it means drinking 1.5-3 litres a day, depending on your size, activity levels, the weather etc. It doesn't have to be just water, though preferably the main part of it will be.

ACTION: Pay attention to your pee when you go! Don't just flush. If it's looking dark you probably need to drink more water. Always get checked if there are any signs of blood.

Staying hydrated will help our energy levels, clear thinking and help avoid hormonal water retention.

Sugar laden fizzy drinks or flavoured coffees are loaded with sugar so stay away. So-called diet drinks contain *sweeteners that have been shown to support the growth of unhealthy gut bacteria* so steer clear[lxiv]. That includes those flavoured waters.

If you struggle with plain water, put a slice of lemon or lime in it, or some other fruit. Caffeinated drinks like tea and coffee are fine in moderation, and preferably not taken from mid-afternoon onwards to avoid sleep disruption. Steer totally clear of the canned energy drinks, they will not do you any health favours at all.

Get acquainted with some herbal teas (not fruit teas with sweetness added), that way you can have a variety of hot drinks that don't spike your blood sugar or frazzle you with caffeine.

Alcohol is mostly *sugar with added toxins* that force your liver to work harder and messes with your hormones, so moderation here is key. If you are really out of balance and struggling with hormonal issues, then maybe give it a miss altogether for a while. Either way, drinking in moderation on the whole is considered as *one drink, occasionally two*, in an evening. It's not nothing all week and then a whole bottle of wine or four gins.

If you do go out and party or have a special event, make a point of steering clear for a while. If you are someone who waits for wine o'clock each day, or is feeling the need to pour a drink every night, it's time to consider your relationship with alcohol.

We all know it's addictive, and most addictions are really started by trying to fulfil a need that's not being met. So if that's you, where the holiday habit of drinking every day has kind of carried on to make it the norm, or you notice yourself really wanting that first drink of the evening, it's time to take a step back.

If it's the symbolism of pouring that drink meaning 'it's time to relax and here's your reward for being a good adult today', then substitute it. These days there are some vastly improving non-alcoholic beers and spirits compared to what there used to be. Pour yourself a can of 0% beer into a glass and sit back. Pour a (naturally low in sugar) tonic into a glass and add the lime. Maybe try one of those pretend spirits. If you can get past that moment of wanting the alcohol by swapping out the alcohol but keeping the symbolism of rewarding yourself , then that's ok.

But do take time to evaluate why you are feeling the need to pour that drink in the first place. And don't be scared to seek help if required. There are plenty of anonymous ways to seek help.

ACTION: Ask yourself honestly how much you've had to drink in the last week, the last fortnight or month. If it's above the recommended 14 units a week (6 glasses of 13% strength wine, 6 pints 4% beer or 14 measures of 25ml spirits) then it's too much. How can you substitute these? Reflect on why you are drinking.

For the sake of balancing your hormones, *do try a total break from alcohol at least a few times a year*. Most of us manage this for at least 9 months when pregnant. Funny how when it's for something that's not ourselves, we can do it. Re-read the section on finding your why if you need something to focus on to do this.

If you've ever done one of these month long challenges you'll know how a month without booze can lead to: better sleep, clearer skin, more energy.

Taken direct from the Priory (an addiction rehabiliation clinic) website are some stats about what a month alcohol free can do for you:

- £89 better off (that's based on not having 24 x 175ml glasses of wine in a month, so for some this will be more)
- 3840 calories less
- Liver function recovered (hormonal balance, improved energy, better vitamin storage)
- 15% loss of liver fat (you really don't want fatty liver)
- Better looking skin
- Reduced blood pressure
- Stomach lining improved
- Sleep improved
- 72% are more mindful about their drinking of the next 6 months.

MOVE:

"Life is like riding a bicycle, to keep your balance you must keep moving." Albert Einstein

We all know we are meant to exercise for health. But because of many of the reasons mentioned in previous chapters, most of us don't do enough. The UK government recommends a MINIMUM of 150 moderately active minutes a week, such as walking, cycling, swimming or, 75 mins of more intense activity like running or sport. Children are advised to be active for an hour a day.

Depressingly, 40% of UK women do not meet these minimum exercise requirements and terrifyingly, 85% of girls (and 75% of boys) are not getting enough exercise[lxv]. Things are so bad that our sedentary lifestyles are now considered up there with smoking as to how damaging it is for our well being.

However, merely pounding out an hour at the gym if the remaining 23 hours of our day are mostly on our backsides is not enough to save us. Not if we want to live a healthy thriving life, not just be alive but in poor health.

If we think back to our ancestors, or people living in the Blue Zones, they did not spend their lives doing exercise programmes, their daily lives caused them to move constantly and in such a way that their hearts and brains were nourished.

Our lives today lack movement, and not just movement but diversity of movement. In her book Move Your DNA, Katy Bowman, a biomechanist explains how when we exercise only the muscles we are specifically using, benefit, so if we keep repeating the same run, the same rowing machine, whilst great on one level, the rest of us is left out.[lxvi]

How we move loads each of our cells in different ways and this has an impact on not only our cellular health, but how our joints and organs are loaded and thus age. Our muscle movement helps pump blood in and out of tissues and thus supports the action of the heart in circulating our blood. When we spend the day not moving, our hearts do most of the work[lxvii].

When we spend the day in one position, whether that's sitting or standing, our muscles and ligaments respond by shortening in some places, lengthening in others, which throws the rest of us out of healthy alignment, creating an unhealthy distribution of load on other parts of our bodies.

Sitting for long hours impacts on or gut function, lack of movement doesn't support good flow of blood in our pelvis and thus uterus and ovaries. *In short, driving to work, sitting or standing all day, coming home and sitting on the sofa, is a total health disaster.*

ACTION: Think of your day to day life. Out of a 24 hour day how much are you really moving? And when you do move, how much is in the same forward moving motion, like walking forward, running forward? How often do you reach your arms above your head, squat, stretch in different directions?

So what to do? Definitely don't ditch the gym or exercise classes if you already do them. And if you don't, do try and incorporate them into your life, see the previous chapters on barriers to change and delegation to work out how to fit these into to your life.

But also switch your focus on how to just *move all day long*. Boogie in the kitchen. Get down on the floor and play with the kids, monkey around, work on being able to be in a squat position (this might need to be worked towards in stages if you aren't used to this), *incorporate as much walking into your day as possible*. Get out of your chair every half an hour and move. A lot will depend on the nature of your job, but *think movement*.

Spend as much time outdoors as you can! Not only is being outdoors in nature (even if it's your back garden or the local park) a boost for your mental health, it's getting you out and moving.

For those who are suffering with chronic fatigue type problems, being told to exercise can seem overwhelming. And frankly impossible. So start with where you are at, even if that means sitting on a bench in the garden working on waving your arms around or rotating your ankles. But move. And gently challenge yourself to do a little more. A daily 5 minute walk if you don't currently go for any walks is progress. Try a gentle form of yoga or tai chi.

If you're already an exercise enthusiast, then consider if your muscles would benefit from stretching and lengthening, are you actually very tight and stiff or are you flexible? Excess exercise can also contribute to cortisol issues in the body, so if your workouts are longer than an hour consider mixing it up with gentle yoga or tai chi.

RELAX AND FEED YOUR SOUL:

Knowing how to switch our brains off and relax is critical for our physical and mental health. Our thoughts have a direct impact on our physical responses.

Try this: take your pulse. Note how many beats per minute it is. Now sit there and think about something you find really stressful or are worried about. Take your pulse again. Chances are, that just by thinking about something stressful your heart rate sped up.

Now focus on something super relaxing. Imagine yourself floating on a soft fluffy cloud with your body soft and relaxed. Feel the calm and joy all around you. Breathe slowly and deeply. Then take your pulse again. Has it gone down?

Without thinking about it we do this to ourselves with our thoughts all day long. It impacts our blood pressure, heart rate, blood sugar and hormonal balance. So learning how to calm the worry in our minds is crucial.

Some people seem to manage this with ease. They simply decide not to think about the things that bother them and focus on what brings them happiness or contentment. Amazing right? This is a real skill, but it's one that can be cultivated.

The more we practise choosing our own thoughts the more we can actively switch off from the ones that bother us. And the more we can observe our thoughts calmly without panic and fear.

Learning to be truly present in the moment is a big step towards this, given that most of what we worry about is in the future. If you struggle with anxiety and worry, then signing up to a mindfulness class is something that is highly recommended. (And if anxiety becomes constant or severe do seek help from your doctor).

Reminding ourselves of the basics in moments of stress can be helpful. Try saying to yourself "right now I am *safe*, I am not in danger, *I am in control* of what happens. I can seek help and support if I don't know how to proceed." Then *breathe slowly and deeply* so your belly rises and falls.

ACTION: Next time you are worrying about something. Take a moment to breathe deeply, and try the following. Say to yourself, "right now I am choosing not to think about x. I will return to thinking about it after I have done the

other things I need to do. Right now, I'm focusing on playing with my child/replying to work emails/preparing dinner" and then do your best to throw yourself fully into the present moment. It's not easy, and you'll likely have to repeat this many times to get even a few moments mental peace.

BREATHE

Learning to simply take the time to breathe fully is one of the best things we can do to calm ourselves. How many of us only breathe with the top part of our lungs? Watch a baby or a dog or cat breathing, their belly rises and falls.

When we belly breathe, we activate the vagus nerve that stimulates the release of calming chemicals throughout the body. You can do this anywhere, anytime. Sitting in a meeting, at traffic lights, on the loo! Get into the habit of *slow belly breathing several times a day* and you will notice your general sense of calm improving.

However, it's not just managing how we feel in a moment of worry that's important. It's choosing to take the time to *actively relax* and allow our bodies to go into a state of relaxation and calm. Given how many of us are running around in a state of chronic stress, we desperately need this respite to lower our stress hormones and rebalance us.

Making time for the activities you love that help you switch off is not something to be treated as an after-thought, but as something vitally important for self-care. Reading, listening to music, gardening, walking the dog, sewing, knitting, crafting, painting, all of these things can help us unwind.

Get regular treatments that help your body and mind rebalance, such as acupuncture (from a professionally trained acupuncturist, preferably member of the British Acupuncture Council) or massage. This will help your body and mind let go of stress and worry and allow clear thinking.

Taking time to think about *positive things* in our lives is also helpful. Cultivating a gratitude practice can help us reset our brains (it quite literally changes our molecular structure) away from all that is not right to all that is going well and is said to boost our sense of well-being and relaxation.

One of my favourite ways to quieten my busy brain is to think of all the things in my life for which I am grateful. Or when something is going wrong during the day, ask myself *what else is going right*, so as to keep the one bad thing from ruining the whole day. There are numerous studies into gratitude which show us that it helps improve our sleep, lower our anxiety and depression and improve our level of exercise.[lxviii]

ACTION: Each morning and each evening, try and list three things for which you are grateful. It doesn't have to big things, even the small things, like seeing the first snow drops in winter, or for having had time to sit quietly with a mug of tea count.

It's not about being an annoying positive Polly and denying your other feelings such as anger, frustration, jealousy etc., but about *owning* them, the good and the bad.

As mentioned previously, in Chinese Medicine the source of most ill health is the emotions. The issue isn't having the emotions, *it's when they stay stuck* within us or *aren't acknowledged*. It takes an awful lot of physical and mental energy to hold onto anger, grief, sadness, frustration. It's exhausting to stay in a constant state of joy. Our bodies feel and respond to these emotions in a very real way, directly impacting our health.

Our emotions are meant to come and go. In terms of managing stress, managing our feelings that arise in the face of difficulty is crucial. Have you noticed how when you get cut up driving the car, on a day you are in a good calm place you sigh, call them a numpty and let it go, but on a day when you're already frazzled, you end up yelling and shouting and feeling really angry and aggressive towards the other driver?

The difference isn't what the driver of the car did, it's where your emotions were already at. Being able to name and own the emotions you have is a crucial way to be able to let go of them and the unpleasant stressful feelings that they bring with them.

The fertility acupuncturist Chris Axelrad, describes an exercise he uses with his fertility patients to help them let go of stuck emotions/energy that could be better used elsewhere in the body:

> He starts by getting them to relax. Then think of a situation that has upset them. Then to visualise the moment their feelings arose. He gets them to name the feelings, be that anger, frustration, fear, jealousy, hurt,

whatever. And *here's the crucial bit*, he gets them to say: "I am feeling [name of feeling]. As the creator of this [name of feeling], I choose to create joy and inner peace instead." Then asks them to really try and create a sense of joy and peace within themselves. [lxix]

I really suggest you try this exercise. Naming an emotion takes the mystery and fear out of it. *Owning it reminds us we are in charge of our feelings*, and choosing joy and peace is again another way of putting us back in charge of our own thoughts.

ACTION: Do the above exercise right now. Now observe how your whole body and mind feels completely different. You can do this exercise anytime you notice feelings that contribute to your sense of stress or overwhelm.

> *"You don't have to quash all the negative emotions that you happen to feel. What you have to do is to teach yourself to generate the emotions you do want to feel on a consistent basis."* Brendon Buchard

Meditation is another practice that helps us switch off the stress and manage what life throws at us with greater ease. In terms of Put Yourself First, this is up there on the list with prioritising sleep, ditching sugar and eating more veg and it's vital this is one of the top items on your daily to do list.

It doesn't have to take long. It can be as simple as *two minutes belly breathing whilst focussing your mind on your breath*. You can do this anywhere. Waiting for a meeting to start. By yourself in the toilet cubicle at work. Sat at your desk. Or it can be a longer practice.

Some people find an app helpful, my personal favourite is the *Calm app* as it's got a mix of shorter and longer mediations, some with different themes. With a pair of headphones you can listen to this whilst on the bus or train (but never when you are driving!). A theme I particularly like to work on is the idea of self-compassion or *loving kindness*.

If we truly learn to treat ourselves with love and compassion, this will filter through into everything we do, and make our life more joyful. Many studies now demonstrate how powerful meditation is for lowering cortisol, lowering blood pressure, managing pain, reducing anxiety and stress, improving concentration, helping fight addiction and just become more self-aware of where we are at in ourselves.[lxx]

CHEMICAL EXPOSURE:

All the chemicals we are exposed to cumulatively add up to disrupt our hormones. In fact, constant exposure to hormone-disrupting chemicals is widely believed (along with excess sugar intake and lack of exercise) to be behind the reason more and more girls are starting their periods earlier and suspected to be part of the cause of the rise in many cancers, insulin resistance, diabetes and other metabolic disorders. They have been linked to fertility issues and diminished ovarian reserve.[lxxi]

We are bombarded daily with a cocktail our bodies are just not meant to deal with and whilst we can't eradicate everything we can minimise our exposure. It is impossible to say what interactions are occurring when the different chemicals combine together in our bodies.

Whilst EU testing and safety regulations have banned the worst offenders, it is clear that many chemicals we currently use are still undergoing testing, and it's not been possible to test the cumulative effect of different cocktails of chemicals we use day after day, year after year. Or how one chemical causes another to have an even stronger effect or releases a previously contained substance.[lxxii]

There is a serious lack of information out there, and whilst things that have been positively found to be problematic have been banned, there are many more chemicals still legally used that are suspected to be endocrine disrupters, but as yet lack enough evidence for a ban to be imposed. All these chemicals have a huge impact on our bodies and environment and some don't break down easily meaning levels rise and rise around us.

To minimise exposure:

- Avoid using plastic where possible, especially heating it with food or drink in. Replace drinks bottles with stainless steel. Coffee mugs with glass or steel (some bamboo products have been found to contain formaldyhyde).

- Around the home, switch to more eco-friendly brands for cleaning products. Or even look up old fashioned methods such as vinegar and baking soda! Exposure to cleaning products can be as bad as smoking.[lxxiii]

- And as for what we put on our skin through deodorants, fragrance, shampoos, conditioners, body creams, soaps, make up, fake tans, hair dye, nail products, try and find products with as few ingredients as possible and with as few chemicals as possible. Luckily more brands are making a move in this direction, but become a label-reader.

KNOW YOUR NUMBERS

If we want to be the ones in charge of our own health and well-being, there are some key things we should all know in relation to where we are at with our health.

YOUR WAIST: Much more important than the exact figure on weighing scales is our waist measurement. Our waist tells us where we are at with the unhealthy fat that can accumulate on our bellies leading to hormonal imbalance, systemic inflammation, heart disease, diabetes etc. The more well-known measurement of dividing height by weight, or BMI, is a less accurate measure of health. After all, you can have someone whose height and weight falls into the healthy range, but if you look at their body shape, and they have skinny little legs but have a load of belly fat, they're, not healthy at all.

The simplest way of knowing what your waist should measure for health, is to halve your height.[lxxiv] So for example, if you are 5ft4 inches your waist shouldn't be above 32inches.

You can also look at dividing your waist measurement by your hip measurement to get your Waist-Hip Ratio. As a woman, your ratio for health is 0.80 or below. 0.81-85 is moderate risk and anything above 0.85 is considered high risk.

If your waist falls into an unhealthy range then it's a sign your blood sugar, stress levels, hormones and activity levels are not ideal.

YOUR HBA1C blood result. This measures how much glucose bonded to your haemoglobin in the last three months and gives us an idea of your average blood sugar control. If you have a waist measurement that is not ideal, or find yourself struggling with low blood sugar dips, constant thirst, feelings of exhaustion etc., you should have this done.

The result is broken down into ranges, normal less than 6%, pre diabetic 6 to 6.4%, and anything above 6.4% is considered diabetic. However, as with many reference ranges, what is classed as normal is different to what is ideal and studies show that for optimal health, it should really fall in the 4.6% to 5.3% range. There is evidence that in non-diabetic people, for each 1% rise above 4.6% the risk of cardiovascular disease doubles[lxxv]. So ask for a HBA1c every year, and if your own doctor won't do it, you can have it done privately.

Your fasting blood glucose: The normal range is usually considered to be less than 99 mg/dl, 100-125 is considered pre-diabetic, 126 upwards is diabetic. As with HBA1c, what is classed as normal isn't always optimal and those with numbers in the 90s can often go on to be diabetic a decade later, so ideally it would be in the 80s.[lxxvi]

Vitamin D levels: many of us are deficient in Vitamin D. We need vitamin D for good bone health, but it also plays a role in ensuring cell growth is normal, thyroid health, neuromuscular and immune function and reducing inflammation. For good health our levels should be between 50-100 nmol/L. (Vitamin D factsheet National Institutes of Health)

There are many other blood tests, vitamin and mineral levels that we could look at, but these are the very basics of which you should be aware.

In a perfect world, we would all have a functional medicine assessment of vitamins, minerals, inflammatory markers, gut health, various fatty acids. This could then give us targeted individual advice on tweaking our health to be as well as possible. If this is something you are interested in doing contact the Institute of Functional Medicine.

Many people ask if we should take *supplements*. Ideally, if we get our diets right we shouldn't need to, and getting what we need from our food is always preferable to any supplement. But where we are tackling stress, or depleted and deficient states, vitamin supplements can be helpful, if, *they are good quality*.

Much of what is sold on the high-street, passes straight through us without doing much good at all. If supplements are needed then being able to approach a company where you can actually ask a qualified nutritionist about their products is a good start, and the products being made from food-derived rather than synthetic vitamins will also be better. My personal choice would be the company Wild Nutrition.

But as with everything, if you already have a diagnosed health condition or are taking medications, *don't supplement without checking with your doctor or pharmacist*.

Taking supplements does not excuse us from putting the effort in with what we eat or do.

CONCLUSION:

As you can see, nourishing yourself is about all that we put onto and into our bodies *and* minds. The suggestions in this chapter are clearly not exhaustive, but are designed to get you thinking about the concepts of each aspect of nourishing yourself so that you can apply it to your life in a way that speaks to you and aligns with your vision of how you want your life to be. All the suggestions are designed to enhance your ability to thrive, not just survive.

CHAPTER 8: PROJECT SELF:

"Changing our behaviour is the single most important step we can take to prevent and reverse chronic disease." Chris Kresser

What better way to finish this busy woman's guide to thriving not surviving, than to help you create Project Self. Your mission, should you choose to accept, is to *make yourself your own project.*

Now that you understand more about how your body works and the different key elements that contribute to your health, you understand your why, how what you think and believe impacts you, and how to create the space in your life for YOU to be priority, you are ready to take this challenge.

If you want to take this further and engage a health coach to support you in this project, get in touch.

Start by identifying which area of self-care in your life is your weakest link, if it helps, score yourself out of 10, 1 meaning you are totally out of balance and not meeting basic needs, and 10 being you have it down to a fine art.

Your Put Yourself First categories of self-care are:

> Sleep
> Food
> Relaxation (physical and mental)
> Exercise and movement
> Strong social and practical support network

Which has your lowest score?

Target this first. If there are two or three equally low scoring categories, start with the one you feel most excited and motivated to tackle first.

Go grab a pen and paper/tablet and take the time to really think and answer the following:

What would it look like to you if you got a high score? Visualise how your life would be if you were doing better in this category? What would you look like? What would day to day life be like? What other areas would naturally start to improve as a result?

Now look at what you are currently doing. *How far away from your ideal is it?*

Why do you think this is? Is it previous lack of knowledge? Time? How your day is structured?

What are your limiting beliefs around this? How can you rewrite them?

What barriers are there that you can see currently preventing you from your ideal? These can be practical (e.g., money, support), or in your mind (thoughts, fears).

How can you *overcome* each of these barriers? Do you need help or is it something that can be tackled fairly easily? If you need help, is it with knowledge? Or practical?

How can you take a totally *fresh approach* to this area of your life?

What do people who do this well do? Who inspires you?

Do take the time to really reflect on the above questions. Talk them through with someone close to you, or someone whose opinion you trust and will speak honestly. Then, once you feel you have really unpicked the issues, move on to the following:

What would you like your goal in this area of self-care to be?

What *support or resources* do you have to achieve your goal? These can be practical and emotional.

What is the first step you could take this week to move towards your goal?

When are you going to do it, which day? How? Be precise.

How are you going to hold yourself accountable to doing this? Are you going to write it down in a journal, tell a partner or friend you are trying to do this?

Once you've taken your first step, what will the next one be?

Who will be your cheerleaders in going for this? Who will you turn to when finding it hard?

By what date in the future would you like to be able to say you are scoring highly on this goal? Be realistic.

What would be a mid-point to your goal, both date and what you would like to have achieved?

If you hit an obstacle or it just doesn't happen on a given day or week, how will you react? How will you pick yourself up or restart?

> "Remember how far you've come, not just how far you have to go. You are not where you want to be, but neither are you where you used to be." Carmel Farnan, British Mindfulness Academy

How can you celebrate each time you reach a milestone?

How will you ensure your new behaviours become your new habits?

KEEP GOING!

Once you have really worked on one area, start again at the beginning and re-score your categories of self-care. It wouldn't be surprising if once you've worked on one your scores on other areas of your life improve. Then, pick your next lowest category and start this process again. Use the handy self-care planner chart below and the veg challenge chart seen earlier to help you keep aspects of self-care on track.

Remember behaviour and lifestyle change is a process. It takes time. Neither is it usually a straight path. But keep at it. You deserve to feel amazing.

And above all, enjoy it! Enjoy the process of change. Live in the present moment. Enjoy getting excited about new ideas, about seeing how differently you can feel, becoming more self-aware. Get used to having time to prioritise yourself being your new normal. Relish feeling better! Enjoy being inspired by other women who have done these things, believe you can be one of them. Believe you deserve to Put Yourself First, to live your best life and thrive!!

> "Let us LOVE ourselves so fiercely that when others see us they know exactly how it should be done." Rudy Francisco

Weekly Self-Care Planner

	Monday	Tuesday	Wednesday	Thursday	Friday	Saturday	Sunday
Wake-Up Time							
Exercise Time							
Meditation / Mindfulness Time							
Time Out Time							
Bed Time							

FURTHER HELP AND RESOURCES:

If you've enjoyed reading this book or found it helpful I'd be ever so grateful if you could leave a review on Amazon!

To find out more about the Women's Health Coaching, online courses or speaking events that Marianne Killick offers please visit www.mariannekillick.com

To find a professionally trained acupuncturist: British Acupuncture Council visit: www.acupuncture.org.uk

For Nutritional Therapists: British Association of Nutritional and Lifestyle Medicine visit: www.bant.org.uk

For Functional Medicine information or practitioners visit the Institute of Functional Medicine: www.ifm.org

For relationship counselling: Relate: www.relate.org.uk

For mental health support: MIND: www.mind.org.uk

For advice on diabetes: Diabetes UK: www.diabetes.org.uk

If you have concerns re your drinking: Drink Aware: www.drinkaware.co.uk

For any practitioners, therapists or services that you engage always check levels of study and qualifications and membership of professional bodies.

If you'd like to read further from any of the authors mentioned or referenced in the book please see the References section.

ACKNOWLEDGEMENTS

With massive thanks to my husband Russ, who has shown the ultimate commitment to teamwork to allow me to turn this book into reality. And thanks to our children for their tolerance of Mummy being immersed more than usual. Thanks to my Mum for keeping the children amused when needed. To Lauren at So Brand Creative for your amazing vision with regards to your artwork. To Heidi from Setchfield VA Services for your practical, efficient and timely support. To Luke, my domestic fairy godmother and cleaner extraordinaire who keeps us organised and calm. To my friend David and my friend Aarti, for their editing prowess. To Jo Bevilacqua and all the women at The Unique Mumpreneur for believing in me and encouraging me to follow my dreams. THANK YOU ALL.

REFERENCES

[i] Brown, Brene, Dare to Lead – Brave work, tough conversations, whole hearts. Vermillion 2018. P158

[ii] Brigid Schulte, "A woman's greatest enemy? A lack of time to herself." Article published in The Guardian, 21 July 2019.

[iii] Ofcom.org.uk Online Nation 2019 report

[iv] Ofcom.org.uk A decade of Digital Dependency 2 August 2018

[v] Bright Horizons Modern Family Index 2017

[vi] Gottschalik, S "Why You Should Spend Your Time Doing Nothing According to Science Published on Livescience.com on 31 May 2018

[vii] Duhigg, C., The Power of Habit – Why we do what we do and how to change Random House 2013, p 85-93

[viii] Dispenza, Joe, Dr, You Are The Placebo - Making your mind matter, Hay House 2014 p105

[ix] Dispenza, Op.Cit p 113-121

[x] Dweck, Carol Dr., Mindset - Changing the way you think to fulfil your potential, Robinson 2017

[xi] Esfahani Smith, E., The Power of Meaning - The True Route to Happiness. Penguin Random House, 2017 p 94

[xii] Esfahani Smith OpCit, p41

[xiii] Woods, W., Good Habits, Bad Habits – The Science of Making Positive Changes That Stick, Macmillan 2019

[xiv] Duhigg Op Cit

[xv] Duhigg Op Cit., Chapter 5

[xvi] Duhigg OpCit., p142-143

[xvii] Wood. W. OpCit

[xviii] Wood, W., Op Cit

[xix] Buettner talking at minutes 30-32 of the Podcast 67 19th June 2019 of Feel Better Live More with Dr Chatterjee

[xx] Duhigg, C., OpCit

[xxixxi] Woods, W., OpCit

[xxii] Buettner, D., The Blue Zones (2nd Edition) - 9 Lessons for Living Longer from the people who've lived the longest, National Geographic 2012

[xxiii]Coulson, J. The Secret to Magic Mornings? Put the kids to work. Article in The New York Times 25 April 2018.

[xxiv] Taylor, S., Tend and Befriend – Behavioural Bases of Affilaition Under Stress, Current Directions in Psychological Science 2006 Vol 15 No6 273-277

[xxv] Yano, J,M., Yu, K., Donaldson GP, et al.., Indigenous bacteria from the gut microbiota regulate host serotonin biosynthesis, in Cell. 2015:161(2):264-276. Doi:10.1016/j.cell.2015.02.047

[xxvi] Valero, J., Paris, I., Sierra, A., Lifestyle Shapes the Dialogue between environment, microglia and adult neurogenesis. ACS Chem.Neurosci. 2016, 7, 4, 442-453 14th March 2016 https://doi.org/10.1021/acschemneuro.6b00009

[xxvii]Kelton Tremellen, Naeema Syedi, Sze Tan & Karma Pearce (2015) Metabolic endotoxaemia – a potential novel link between ovarian inflammation and impaired progesterone production, Gynecological Endocrinology, 31:4, 309-312, DOI: 10.3109/09513590.2014.994602

[xxviii]Balter, L. J. T., Bosch, J. A., Aldred, S., Drayson, M. T., Veldhuijzen van Zanten, J. J. C. S., Higgs, S., Raymond, J., Mazaheri, A. (2019). Selective effects of acute low-grade inflammation on human visual attention. *NeuroImage*, 202, 116098. doi:https://doi.org/10.1016/j.neuroimage.2019.116098

[xxix] Science Mag "Link Between Inflammation and mental sluggishness shown in new study" 15th November 2019.

[xxx] Hirschberg, S; Gisevius, B.,;Duscha, A., Haghikia, A. Implications of Diet and the Gut Microbiome in Neuroinflammatory and Neurodegenerative Diseases Int. J. Mol. Sci. 2019, 20, 3109

[xxxi] Castellino A M, "Diet could influence immunotherapy response via microbiome" Medscape Medical News, 4th March 2019

[xxxii] Quote from Dr Mark Hyman, TED Talk 26 July 2018.

[xxxiii]Chen JT, Kotani K., Oral Contraceptive Therapy increases oxidative stress in pre-menopausal women. Int J Prev Med. 2012 Dec;3(12):893-6

[xxxiv] Joseph D F and Whirledge S, Stress and the HPA Axis: Balancing homeostasis and fertility, Journal of Molecular Sciences Int J Mol Science. 2017 Oct; 18(10): 2224)

[xxxv] Szmelskyj & Aquilina, L., Acupuncture for IVF and assisted reproduction – An integrated approach to treatment and management Churchill-Livingstone Elsevier 2015 P32-33

[xxxvi] Joseph D F and Whirledge S, Stress and the HPA Axis: Balancing homeostasis and fertility, Journal of Molecular Sciences Int J Mol Science. 2017 Oct; 18(10): 2224)

[xxxvii] Kelton Tremellen, Naeema Syedi, Sze Tan & Karma Pearce (2015) Metabolic endotoxaemia – a potential novel link between ovarian inflammation and impaired progesterone production, Gynecological Endocrinology, 31:4, 309-312, DOI: 10.3109/09513590.2014.994602

[xxxviii] Drummond J, The Pregnenelone Steal in Module 25 of Women's Health Coach course, Integrative Women's Health Institute

[xxxix] Sky News, Weight Gain in 20s to Late 40s linked to early death. 17 October 2019

[xl] LaMotte, S., Lifestyle Changes Improved cognition in people at risk for alzheimers, study shows. Published on CNN 30 Oct 2019, discusses recent study published in the journal Alzheimers and Dementia, the Journal of the Alzheimers Association.

[xli] Jackson, G, The female problem: how male bias in medical trials ruined women's health Published in The Guardian 13th November 2019

[xlii] Menolascino, M., MD, Heart Solution for Women - A proven programme to prevent and reverse heart disease. Harper One, 2019

[xliii] Axelrad, Chris, Awakening The Seed - The New, Simplified, Proven Path to Pefect Egg Quality, Optimal Fertility and Healthy Babies, Axelrad Clinic 2019.p134

[xliv] Drummond J, LECTURE Module 25 of Women's Health Coach course, Integrative Women's Health Institute

[xlv] Wilcox, A., Dunson, D., Baird, D,D., The Timing of the "fertile window" in the menstrual cycle: day specific estimates of a prospective study BMJ, 2001, January 6; 322(7277):28

[xlvi] Hill, M., Period Power - harness your hormones and get your cycle working for you. Green Tree 2019

[xlvii] Weschler, T, Taking Charge of Your Fertility, Harper Collins 2003

[xlviii] Mitra, A Dr, The Gynae Geek - Your no-nonsense guide to 'down there' healthcare, Thorsons 2019

[xlix] Sleep Council "Great British Bedtime Report 2017" www.sleepcouncil.org.uk

[l] Hamilton John, How Deep Sleep May Help The Brain Clear Alzheimers Toxins, 31 Oct 2019, published on npr.org, discusses the research published in the journal Science

[li] Buettber, D. OpCit

[lii] [lii] 2017 healthsurvey.hscic.gov.uk

[liv] Wighton, K., Eating More Fruits and Vegetables May Prevent Millions of Premature Deaths. Published on imperial.ac.uk on 23 Feb 2017 discussing the research by scientists from Imperial College London published in the International Journal of Epidemiology.

[lv] Sandolu, A, Largest Microbiome study weighs in on our gut health 15th May 2018 published on Medical News Today.com discussing the research findings of the American Gut Project

Serin Y and Acar Tek N, Effect of Circadian Rhythm on Metabolic Processes and the Regulation of Energy Balance. Annals of Nutrition and Metabolism, 2019: 74:322-330[lvi]

[lvii] Panda, Satchin, The Circadian Code- Lose weight, supercharge your energy and sleept well every night. Vermilion 2018

[lviii] Panda, OpCit.

[lix] Wilkinson et al, 2020, Ten Hour Time Restricted Eating Reduces Weight, Blood Pressure, and Atherogenic Lipids in Patients with Metabolic Syndrome. Cell Metabolism 31, 1-13, January 7 2020 https://doi.org/10.1016/j.cmet.2019.11.004

[lx]Brogan, Kelly, MD A Mind of Your Own- the truth about depression and how women can heal their bodies to reclaim their lives. Thorsons 2016 p90

[lxi] Niland, B., and Brooks, C. D., Health Benefits and Advserse Effects of A Gluten Free Diet in Non Coeliac Disease Patients, Gastroenterol Hepatol (NY), 2018 Feb: 14 (2):82-91

[lxii]Wahls, T, MD The Wahls Protocol - a radical new way to treat all chronic autoimmune conditions using paleo principles, Penguin 2014

[lxiii] Kresser, C., The Gluten-Thyroid Connection, posted on chriskresser.com 16 March 2019

[lxiv] (J Suez R.T. al., "Artificial Sweeteners Induce Glucose Intolerance by Altering the Gut Microbiota." Nature, 514, no 7521 (October 9, 2014): 181-86, doi; 10.1038/nature13793)

[lxv] (Gallagher, J, Global Epidemic of Childhood Inactivity, BBC.co.uk 22 November 2019)
.

[lxvi] Bowman, K MS, Move Your DNA - restore your health through natural movement , Short Run Press 2014

[lxvii] Bowman, K MS, Move Your DNA - restore your health through natural movement , Short Run Press 2014

[lxviii] . (Brown, J, "Neuroscience reveals: This is how gratitude literally rewires your brain to be happier." Published on realfarmacy.com

[lxix] Axelrad, Op.Cit., p141-142.

[lxx] Thorpe, Matthew, 12 Science-Based Benefits of Meditation, published on Healthline, 5 July 2017. Each of these points is linked to research studies within the articles, so to read more, follow the links in the original article.)

[lxxi] Ripamonti, E, Allifranchini, E, Todeschi, S, Bocchietto, E, Endocrine Disruptors by Topical Consumer Products, Cosmetics 2018, 5 (4) 61

[lxxii] Ripamonti, E, Allifranchini, E, Todeschi, S, Bocchietto, E, Endocrine Disruptors by Topical Consumer Products, Cosmetics 2018, 5 (4) 61

[lxxiii] Axe, J Dr, "Home Cleaning Products: Lung Damage Equivalent to Smoking 20 cigarettes a day study says" published 30 Sept 2019 on www.healthyholisticliving.com, the article summarises the findings of research published in the American Journal of Respiratory and Critical Care Medicine.

[lxxiv] Ashwell M, Gibson S Waist-to-height ratio as an indicator of 'early health risk': simpler and more predictive than using a 'matrix' based on BMI and waist circumference BMJ Open 2016;6:e010159. doi: 10.1136/bmjopen-2015-010159

[lxxv] (Selvin E, Coresh J, Golden SH, Brancati FL, Folsom AR, Steffes MW. Glycemic Control and Coronary Heart Disease Risk in Persons With and Without Diabetes: The Atherosclerosis Risk in Communities Study. Arch Intern Med. 2005;165(16):1910–1916.
doi:https://doi.org/10.1001/archinte.165.16.1910

[lxxvi] .Nichols, GA, Hillier TA, Brown, JB, Normal Fasting Plasma Glucose and Risk of Type 2 Diabetes Diagnosis, The American Journal Of Medicine 2008 (02:026)
https://doi.org/10.1016/j.amjmed.2008.02.026